W9-CXJ-441

Activity Pack to Accompany

Medical Terminology Systems

A BODY SYSTEMS APPROACH

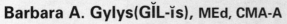

Barbara A. Gylys(GĬL-ĭs), MEd, CMA-A
Professor Emerita
College of Health and Human Services
Medical Assisting Technology
University of Toledo
Toledo, Ohio

Mary Ellen Wedding, MEd, MT(ASCP), CMA, AAPC
Professor of Health Professions
College of Health Science and Human Service
University of Toledo
Toledo, Ohio

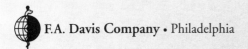
F.A. Davis Company • Philadelphia

F. A. Davis Company
1915 Arch Street
Philadelphia, PA 19103

Last digit indicates print number: 10 9 8 7 6 5 4 3 2 1

Printed in the United States of America.

CONTENTS

Overview v

Suggested Course Outlines 1

Textbook Course Assignments 2
Textbook Course Assignments with TermPlus Software 3

Student- and Instructor-Directed Activities 4

Independent Projects and Oral Reports 4
   Reporting on Current Events (Newspapers, Magazines, Journals) 4
   Accessing Professional Websites 4
   Using Professional Journals 4
Resources for Student- and Instructor-Directed Activities 4
   Technical Journals 4
   Community and Internet Resources 5
   Peer Evaluation Form 6
   Listen-and-Learn Activity Template 7
Clinical Connection Activities 8
   Clinical Connection Activity Answer Key 19
Flowchart Activities 20
   Answer Key for Flowchart Activities 25
Pronunciation and Spelling Activities 26

Supplemental Medical Record Activities 48

Answer Key 89

Crossword Puzzles 117

Answer Key 132

Textbook Medical Record Pronunciations and Answer Key 146

Master Transparencies 166

Overview

You will find the sixth edition of *Medical Terminology Systems: A Body Systems Approach* lives up to its well-established track record of presenting medical word-building principles based on competency-based curricula. *Systems*, 6th ed., is designed with the educational foundation of a textbook-workbook format that complements traditional lecture and classroom teaching as well as distance learning methods. The purpose of the book is to help students learn medical terminology so they can effectively communicate with other members of the health-care team in a confident, professional manner. A variety of pedagogical features will help them develop a strong foundation in medical terminology and broaden their medical vocabulary. Although the study of medical terminology demands hard work and discipline, various self-paced activities offer interest and variety to the learning process.

Beginning with Chapter 2, this edition includes flash-card activities so students can preview, practice, and reinforce word elements presented in the chapter. The DavisPlus icon ![DavisPlus DavisPlus.fadavis.com], found after each Word Elements table, directs students to www.davisplus. fadavis.com/gylys/systems for online flash-card activities focusing on word elements. In addition, a *Listen and Learn Online* activity is available for the medical records included in Chapters 4 through 15. A special icon and instructions prompt the student to visit the DavisPlus website.

All changes in the sixth edition are structured to help in the learning process and improve retention of medical terms. Of the many striking enhancements to this edition are the many new, visually impressive, full-color illustrations. The artwork throughout the book is specifically designed to present accurate and esthetically pleasing representations of anatomical structures, disease conditions, and medical procedures. Illustrations enhance course content in new and interesting ways and help make difficult concepts clear.

The sixth edition continues to present eponyms without showing the possessive form, such as *Bowman capsule, Cushing syndrome,* and *Parkinson disease.* Medical dictionaries as well as the American Association for Medical Transcription and the American Medical Association support these changes.

New to this edition is a summary of common symbols as well as an updated list of "do-not-use" abbreviations. The summaries are found in Appendix B, Common Abbreviations and Symbols.

Each body systems chapter continues to incorporate the most current technological changes in medicine. Educators and practitioners in various health-care disciplines have offered many helpful suggestions for this edition, many of which have been incorporated. A newly developed list of key anatomical and physiological terms, complete with pronunciations and definitions, sets a solid base for the chapter.

Also new to this edition is a body connections section for each body systems chapter. This table identifies the interrelationship of each body system and helps put each system into clear perspective for the student. Diagnostic and therapeutic procedures have also been expanded. Finally, pharmacology information has been edited to include drugs most commonly used in medical treatment. This section continues to provide generic and trade names, along with each drug's therapeutic actions.

The popular basic features found in the previous edition have been expanded and enhanced. Here's a breakdown of those features:

- *Chapter 1* explains the techniques of medical word building using basic word elements.
- *Chapter 2* categorizes major surgical, diagnostic, symptomatic, and grammatical suffixes.
- *Chapter 3* presents major prefixes of position, number and measurement, direction, and other parameters.
- *Chapter 4* introduces anatomical, physiological, and pathological terms as well as combining forms denoting cellular and body structure, body position and direction, and regions of the body. Additional combining forms related to body structure, diagnostic methods, and pathology are also presented. General diagnostic and therapeutic terms are described and provide a solid foundation for specific terms addressed in the body systems chapters that follow.
- *Chapters 5 to 15* are organized according to specific body systems and may be taught in any sequence.

These chapters include key anatomical and physiological terms; anatomy and physiology; body connections; combining forms, suffixes, and prefixes; pathology; diagnostic, symptomatic, and related terms; diagnostic and therapeutic procedures; pharmacology; abbreviations; learning activities; and medical record activities. All activities allow self-assessment and evaluation of competency.

- *Appendix A: Answer Key* contains answers to each learning activity to validate competency and provide immediate feedback for student assessment.
- *Appendix B: Abbreviations* includes an updated, comprehensive list of medical abbreviations and their meanings. It also contains a summary of common symbols as well as an updated list of "do-not-use" abbreviations.
- *Appendix C: Glossary of Medical Word Elements* contains an alphabetical list of medical word elements and their meanings along with page numbers where they are located in the textbook. This appendix employs two methods for word-element indexing—by medical word element and by English term.
- *Appendix D: Index of Genetic Disorders* lists genetic disorders presented in the textbook.
- *Appendix E: Index of Diagnostic Imaging Procedures* contains radiographic and other diagnostic imaging procedures presented in the textbook.
- *Appendix F: Index of Pharmacology* lists medications presented in the textbook.
- *Appendix G: Index of Oncological Terms* includes terms related to oncology presented in the textbook.

■ ■ ■ Supplemental Teaching Aids

A variety of supplemental teaching aids are available free of charge to instructors who adopt the sixth edition of *Medical Terminology Systems: A Body Systems Approach*. When these ancillary products are integrated into your course, they will enhance course content that ensures your students a full curriculum of medical terminology excellence.

INSTRUCTOR'S RESOURCE DISK

The Instructor's Resource Disk (IRD) features many new, innovative instructional aids designed to make teaching medical terminology easier and more effective. The supplemental teaching aids can be used in various educational settings—traditional classroom, distance learning, and independent or self-paced studies. The IRD consists of an Activity Pack, two PowerPoint presentations, an easily retrievable image bank, an Interactive Teaching Tool (ITT), and a Wimba computerized test bank, a powerful, user-friendly test-generation program.

Activity Pack

The Activity Pack* has been expanded to meet today's instructional needs and now includes:

- *Suggested Course Outlines*. Course outlines are provided to help you plan the best method of covering material presented in the textbook. A new, additional course outline is provided for textbooks packaged with *TerminologyPlus*, our completely revised and updated interactive software. Now it will be easy to correlate instructional software with textbook chapters.
- *Student and Instructor-Directed Activities*. These comprehensive teaching aids have been updated and new ones have been added. They provide an assortment of activities for each body system chapter. Activities can be used as required content or as supplemental material. In addition, activities can be assigned as individual or group projects. For group projects, Peer Evaluation Forms have been provided. This edition includes a new Clinical Connection activity and answer key for each chapter.
- *Community and Internet Resources*. This section provides an expanded list of resources, including technical journals, community organizations, and Internet sites to complement course content.
- *Clinical Connection Activities*. These activities provide clinical scenarios that test the student's comprehension of the information presented in each chapter.
- *Flowchart Activities*. The flowchart activities are designed to strengthen the student's comprehension of anatomy and physiology. Using the provided word list, students will complete a flowchart of structures in sequence for each of the physiological processes listed below.
- *Supplemental Medical Record Activities*. The supplemental medical record activities have been updated and include student activities that complement and expand information presented in the body system chapters. As in the textbook, these activities use common clinical scenarios to show how medical terminology is used to document patient care. Medical terms, their pronunciations, a medical record analysis, and an answer key are provided for the supplemental medical records activities. Each medical

---

*The Activity Pack is available in hard copy on request for those who adopt the textbook.

record highlights a specific body system that corresponds to a medical specialty. The medical records can be used for various activities, including oral reports, medical coding, medical transcribing, or individual assignments. All of the authentic medical reports are presented in a two-column style so your students have an opportunity to retype the report in an acceptable one-column format. All of the medical reports are correctly styled in the textbook and can be used as a reference to complete this activity. If you choose to have your students type and format the supplemental medical records in this Activity Pack, you can find correctly formatted versions in the instructional ancillaries section of http://davisplus.fadavis.com/gylys/systems.

In addition, each medical record highlights a specific body system that corresponds to a medical specialty.

- *Textbook Medical Records Activities Pronunciations and Answer Keys.* The sixth edition continues to provide an answer key for the terminology section of medical records presented in selected chapters of the textbook. This answer key is found in the Activity Pack on page 2. It should prove to be a helpful when you discuss the medical record or correct assignments.
- *Crossword Puzzles.* These fun, educational activities are included for each body system chapter. They are designed to reinforce material covered in the chapter and can be used individually or in groups. They can also be used for extra credit or "just for fun." An answer key is included for each puzzle.
- *Master Transparencies.* The transparency pages offer large, clear, black-and-white anatomical illustrations for each body system, which are perfect for making overhead transparencies.

PowerPoint Presentations

Systems, 6th ed., contains four powerful PowerPoint presentations. *Lecture Notes* provides an outline-based presentation for each body system chapter. It consists of a chapter overview, main functions of the body system, and selected pathology, vocabulary, and procedures. Full-color illustrations from the book are included. *MedTerm Workout* is an interactive presentation in which terms drop into view at a click of the mouse. Students can be prompted to say the term aloud, define the term, or provide other feedback before moving to the next term.

Image Bank

New to this edition is a Flash-based image bank that contains all illustrations from the textbook. It is fully searchable and allows users to zoom in and out and

display a JPG image of an illustration that can be copied into a Microsoft Word document or PowerPoint presentation. It is available for instructors who adopt the textbook at http://davisplus.fadavis.com/gylys/systems and on the IRD.

Name that Part is a unique interactive presentation that allows you to guide students in identifying specific parts of a body system. Lastly, the *Interactive Teaching Tool* (ITT) is a brand-new instructional ancillary for use in the classroom. The tool is an Adobe Flash application of images from the book, followed by questions and answers relevant to the illustration. You can zoom in and out of images and test the students' knowledge as you lead discussion of the content. All are available for instructors who adopt the textbook at http://davisplus. fadavis.com/gylys/systems and on the IRD.

Wimba Electronic Test Bank

This edition offers a powerful new test-generating program called Wimba. It enables instructors to create custom-made or randomly generated tests in a printable format from a test bank of more than 1,240 test items. The test bank includes multiple-choice, true-false, and matching questions. Because of the flexibility of the Wimba test-generating program, instructors are able to edit questions in the test bank to meet their specific educational needs. Therefore, if instructors wish to restate, embellish, or streamline questions or change distractors, they can do so with very little effort. Furthermore, they can also add questions to the test bank. The Wimba program requires Windows 95, Windows 98, or Windows NT and is available for Macintosh on request.

DAVISPLUS TEACHING TOOLS

The DavisPlus website (http://davisplus.fadavis.com/ gylys/systems) is a study companion website for *Systems,* 6th ed. It provides activities to accelerate learning and reinforce information presented in each chapter. The DavisPlus icon ![DavisPlus](DavisPlus.fadavis.com) found within the chapters tells students when it is most advantageous to integrate the activities on DavisPlus website into their studies. All online exercises provide instructions for completing the various activities. The multimedia activities available for students on DavisPlus include:

- pronunciations and meanings of newly introduced medical terms from Word Elements tables to improve retention
- flash-card activities for preview and practice to reinforce word elements presented in the chapter
- medical record exercises (including activities in Chapters 4 through 15) that allow students to click highlighted terms in the medical record and hear

their pronunciations and meanings to strengthen understanding of terms

- animations, such as exploration of the pathology of gastroesophageal reflux disease (GERD) or the various stages of pregnancy and delivery, to help students better understand complex processes and procedures
- word search games that present a variety of medical terms to reinforce word recognition and spelling in a fun activity.

AUDIO CD

Some versions of *Systems*, 6th ed., are packaged with an audio CD recording. The CD provides exercises designed to help students strengthen spelling, pronunciation, and understanding of selected medical terms. The audio CD can also be used in beginning transcription and medical secretarial courses. Transcription skills can be developed by typing each word as it is pronounced. After the words are typed, spelling can be corrected by referring to the textbook or a medical dictionary.

TERMPLUS

TermPlus v3.0 is a powerful, interactive CD-ROM program offered with some texts, depending on which version has been selected. TermPlus is a competency-based, self-paced, multimedia program that includes graphics, audio, and a dictionary culled from *Taber's Cyclopedic Medical Dictionary*, 20th edition. Help

menus provide navigational support. The software comes with numerous interactive learning activities, including:

- Anatomy Focus
- Tag the Elements (Drag-and-Drop)
- Spotlight the Elements
- Concentration
- Build Medical Words
- Programmed Learning
- Medical Vocabulary
- Chart Notes
- Spelling
- Crossword Puzzles
- Word Scramble
- Terminology Teaser.

All activities can be graded and the results printed or e-mailed to an instructor. This feature makes the CD-ROM especially valuable as a distance-learning tool because it provides evidence of student drill and practice in various learning activities.

■ ■ ■ *Taber's Cyclopedic Medical Dictionary*

The world famous *Taber's Cyclopedic Medical Dictionary* is the recommended companion reference for this book. Virtually all terms in *Systems* may be found in *Taber's*. In addition, *Taber's* contains etymologies for nearly all main entries presented in this textbook.

Suggested Course Outlines

Medical terminology can be taught in varying lengths of time. One-semester and two-semester courses seem to be the most popular arrangements. A semester usually consists of approximately 15 weeks with a final examination during the 16th week. However, the textbook can be completed in a much shorter period of time. Hospital-based or proprietary school curricula might warrant much less time. The design of this text permits such flexibility, as parts of each chapter can function as a self-tutorial, allowing students to cover course content on their own.

Regardless of the academic time frame, the first four chapters must be mastered because they provide the foundation for medical word building. Thereafter, selection of chapters and extent of coverage presented is at the discretion of each teacher.

In a one-semester course, each chapter is allotted about 1 week to complete the entire book. The design of the book supports a "pick-and-choose" method of assigning work. For example, in addition to assigning all word elements, you may select pathology and abbreviations for testing purposes. In radiology programs, the word elements, pathology, abbreviations, and radiology may be assigned for testing purposes, and so forth. In a one-semester course, testing can be limited to a mid-term and final examination.

Depending on course design, Student- and Instructor-Directed Activities (Activity Pack, pages 8–39) can be integrated within the 15-week period as classroom or group activities or homework assignments. Additional activities are also available in the Activity Pack. In a two-semester course, the outlines provided below can be divided in half, with time expanded for each as needed.

TEXTBOOK COURSE ASSIGNMENTS

The following table provides the textbook course assignment schedule for a one-semester, 15-week course for *Medical Terminology: A Body Systems Approach*, 6th ed., by Barbara Gylys and Mary Ellen Wedding.

Week	Complete (✓)	Textbook Assignment	Student Notes
1–2		Chapter 1: Basic Elements of a Medical Word	
		Chapter 2: Suffixes	
		Chapter 3: Prefixes	
3		Chapter 4: Body Structure	
4		Chapter 5: Integumentary System	
5		Chapter 6: Digestive System	
6–7		Chapter 7: Respiratory System	
		Midterm Examination	
8		Chapter 8: Cardiovascular System	
9		Chapter 9: Blood, Lymph, and Immune Systems	
10		Chapter 10: Musculoskeletal System	
11		Chapter 11: Genitourinary System	
12		Chapter 12: Female Reproductive System	
13		Chapter 13: Endocrine System	
14		Chapter 14: Nervous System	
15		Chapter 15: Special Senses	
		Final Examination	

TEXTBOOK COURSE ASSIGNMENTS WITH TERMPLUS SOFTWARE

The following table provides the course assignment schedule for a one-semester, 15-week course for *Medical Terminology: A Body Systems Approach,* 6th ed., by Barbara Gylys and Mary Ellen Wedding, with TermPlus CD-ROM Interactive Medical Terminology Software by Barbara Gylys and Regina Masters (See page 6).

Depending on course design, Student- and Instructor-Directed Activities (Activity Pack, pages 8–39) can be integrated within the 15-week period as classroom or group activities or homework assignments. Additional activities are also available in the Activity Pack.

Week	✓	Textbook Assignment	✓	TerminologyPlus Assignment	Student Notes
1–2		Chapter 1: Basic Elements of a Medical Word			
		Chapter 2: Suffixes		Suffixes and Prefixes Module	
		Chapter 3: Prefixes			
3		Chapter 4: Body Structure		Body Structure Module	
4		Chapter 5: Integumentary System		Integumentary Module	
5		Chapter 6: Digestive System		Digestive Module	
6–7		Chapter 7: Respiratory System		Respiratory Module	
		Midterm Examination			
8		Chapter 8: Cardiovascular System		Cardiovascular Module	
9		Chapter 9: Blood, Lymph, and Immune Systems		Blood and Lymphatic Module	
10		Chapter 10: Musculoskeletal System		Musculoskeletal Module	
11		Chapter 11: Genitourinary System		Male Reproductive Module Urinary Module	
12		Chapter 12: Female Reproductive System		Female Reproductive Module	
13		Chapter 13: Endocrine System		Endocrine System Module	
14		Chapter 14: Nervous System		Nervous System Module	
15		Chapter 15: Special Senses		Special Senses: Eyes and Ears Module	
		Final Examination			

Student- and Instructor-Directed Activities

The following comprehensive teaching aids are enhanced for this edition. These practical application activities present a platform of course material designed with variety and interest that reinforces the learning process. You can select the activities you feel are appropriate for your course and determine whether they are to be undertaken individually, with peers, or as a group project. If group projects are selected, a Peer Evaluation Form is available on page 6.

■ ■ ■ Independent Projects and Oral Reports

This Activity Pack contains a list of suggested resources for projects and reports. The list contains numerous sources, including journals and websites. (See pages 8–11 of the Activity Pack for this list.)

REPORTING ON CURRENT EVENTS (NEWSPAPER, MAGAZINE, JOURNAL)

Direct the student to an article from the Health and Medicine section of a national newspaper or magazine. The student should prepare an oral presentation, briefly summarizing the issue(s) covered in the article. The summary should identify five key terms from the article that the student can define using *Taber's* or another medical dictionary. As a written component of this assignment, the student may also submit an article summary and a list of key terms with definitions and pronunciations along with a copy of the article.

ACCESSING PROFESSIONAL WEBSITES

Direct the student to the Internet for a professional health organization website, such as the American Academy of Orthopaedic Surgery. Ask the student to download material from the patient education information area and present an oral report on a selected topic. The report should identify five key terms used in the patient education information, including definitions and pronunciations as found in *Taber's*

or another medical dictionary. As a written component of this assignment, the student may also submit a report, including a list of key terms with definitions and pronunciations, as well as a printout of the patient education information found on the website.

USING PROFESSIONAL JOURNALS

Direct the student to identify a professional journal related to the body system being studied. For example, when studying the reproductive system, the student might be directed to the journal *Fertility and Sterility* or to the medical specialty of gynecology. Ask the student to prepare a list of terms found in the article and write the definitions, pronunciations, and any abbreviations found in the article. As an oral report component of this assignment, ask the student to provide the class with a short summary of the journal article by reading and paraphrasing the article's abstract. The student can also photocopy the abstract and underline any words in the abstract that are also found in the key terms list.

■ ■ ■ Resources for Student- and Instructor-Directed Activities

TECHNICAL JOURNALS

The following journals are available from public libraries, academic institutions, and hospitals. Direct your students to professional journals for outside assignments. Here is a brief list of the journals students might select.

American Journal of Hematology
Emergency Medicine
Health Care Management Review
Journal of the American Medical Association
Journal of Nursing

Journal of Clinical Endocrinology and Metabolism
New England Journal of Medicine
Nursing Forum
Nutrition and Cancer
Professional Medical Assistant

COMMUNITY AND INTERNET RESOURCES

Various state and local organizations offer educational information that can be used to supplement classroom instruction. Pamphlets, films, and speakers may be available from state and local societies. Check the phone directory under *Associations* to find organizations available in your community. A rich source of information is also available on the Internet. You might wish to check the resources listed in the table below.

Organization	Internet Address
ALZHEIMER ASSOCIATION	www.alz.org
AMERICAN ACADEMY OF ALLERGY ASTHMA & IMMUNOLOGY	www.aaaai.org
AMERICAN CANCER SOCIETY	www.cancer.org
AMERICAN DENTAL ASSOCIATION	www.ada.org
AMERICAN DIABETES ASSOCIATION	www.diabetes.org
AMERICAN DIETETIC ASSOCIATION	www.eatright.org
AMERICAN LIVER FOUNDATION	www.liverfoundation.org
AMERICAN LUNG ASSOCIATION	www.lungusa.org
AMERICAN RED CROSS	www.redcross.org
ARTHRITIS FOUNDATION	www.arthritis.org
BRAIN INJURY ASSOCIATION OF AMERICA	www.biausa.org
JOHNSON & JOHNSON	www.jnj.com
JUVENILE DIABETES RESEARCH FOUNDATION INTERNATIONAL	www.jdrf.org
MARCH OF DIMES	www.modimes.org
MUSCULAR DYSTROPHY ASSOCIATION	www.mdausa.org
NATIONAL HEMOPHILIA FOUNDATION	www.hemophilia.org
NATIONAL INSTITUTE OF ARTHRITIS AND MUSCULOSKELETAL AND SKIN DISEASES	www.niams.nih.gov
NATIONAL KIDNEY FOUNDATION	www.kidney.org
NATIONAL MULTIPLE SCLEROSIS SOCIETY	www.nmss.org
NATIONAL PARKINSON FOUNDATION, INC.	www.parkinson.org
NATIONAL SCOLIOSIS FOUNDATION	www.scoliosis.org

*A copy of these resources can be distributed to students to complete the directed activities.

PEER EVALUATION FORM

Date: _____   Project Title: _____

Project Member(s): _____

Evaluator's Name: _____

	Possible Points	Points Earned	Comments
Introduction:			
• Topic	5	_____	
• Objectives	5	_____	
Presentation			
• Organization	5	_____	
• Research of Topic	5	_____	
• Clarity of Presentation	5	_____	
• Knowledge of Subject Matter	5	_____	
• Audience Contact	5	_____	
• Creativity/Originality	5	_____	
• Conclusion(s)	5	_____	
Professionalism			
Was the information fully documented with reference?	5	_____	
Were handouts provided and were they appropriate?	5	_____	
Was the presentation at an appropriate level for the audience?	5	_____	

LISTEN-AND-LEARN ACTIVITY TEMPLATE

Use this template to take advantage of the Listen-and-Learn audio CD-ROM.

Chapter title: _____

Objective: **To correctly pronounce and spell the medical terms dictated on the audio CD-ROM. The terms are taken from the Medical Word Elements table in the above-listed chapter.**

Pronunciation Instructions

1. As you listen to the audio CD-ROM, the combining form and its meaning will be presented. Next a medical term that incorporates the combining form and its definition will be presented. Finally, the key term will be repeated, followed by a pause. For example, in the Digestive System chapter, you will hear the following: **gastr/o** means *stomach*. **Gastralgia is a pain in the stomach. Gastralgia (Pause).**

2. During the pause, pronounce the medical term to help you learn its correct pronunciation. We also recommend that you follow along in your book so you can see the combining forms and key terms in print as you hear them pronounced.

3. Last, place a red checkmark next to the word in your book if you have pronounced the word correctly. Highlight words you did not pronounce correctly, and repeat the activity until you are proficient.

After you have learned the correct pronunciation for the medical terms on the CD, you can enhance your spelling skills by completing the spelling activity below.

Spelling Instructions

1. Listen to the audio CD-ROM for the combining form and its meaning. Next you'll hear a medical term that incorporates the combining form and the definition of the medical term. Finally, the medical term will be repeated again, followed by a pause.

2. During the pause, write the key term on a numbered sheet of paper. For example, in the Digestive System chapter, you'll hear the following: **gastr/o** means *stomach*. **Gastralgia is a pain in the stomach. Gastralgia (Pause).**

3. Last, check your spelling by comparing the spelling of each term with the terms in the appropriate section of the textbook.

Note: **You can begin to develop transcription skills by modifying the spelling instructions. Instead of writing the key terms on a numbered sheet of paper, use a word-processing program to type the words as they are dictated.**

Your name: _____

Competency Verification

Use a calculator to compute your score.

Number of correct pronunciations: _____ ÷ number of words dictated = _____ %

Number of correct spellings: _____ ÷ number of words dictated = _____ %

Staple a copy of your spelling word list to this document.

Clinical Connection Activity—Chapter 5: Integumentary System

alopecia	ecchymosis	petechia
antihistamine	eschar	scabies
cellulitis	metastasis	tuberculosis
debridement	parasiticide	urticaria

Complete the statements by selecting a medical term from the list above.

1. Alex H., a 5th grade student, is sent home by the school nurse after she notices pediculosis while assessing his height and weight. The nurse instructs Alex's mother to wash his hair with permethrin, a _____.

2. The physician informs a 32-year-old woman with breast cancer about the adverse effects of chemotherapy. The woman is most concerned with the hair loss, or _____, that commonly occurs with chemotherapy.

3. The physician informs John K., a 54-year-old construction worker with a history of colon cancer, that malignant cells from his primary tumor spread to his lungs. This process is called _____.

4. Kelsey A., a chef at a local gourmet restaurant, suffers a severe burn injury involving the epidermis and part of the dermis. Within a few days a scab called a(n) _____ forms over the injured site.

5. A patient is admitted to the hospital with swelling, warmth, redness, and pain of the right lower extremity. The physician suspects _____ , a diffuse, acute infection of the skin and subcutaneous tissue.

6. A patient develops acute shortness of breath 12 hours after suffering a left femur fracture. Suspecting fat embolism, you assess the patient's skin and note minute, pinpoint hemorrhages under the patient's skin, known as _____.

7. The infection control nurse places a patient on contact precautions to protect staff from a contagious skin disease transmitted by the itch mite. This condition is commonly known as _____.

8. The employee health nurse is performing annual Mantoux tests on the hospital staff. This intradermal test screens for _____.

9. Anna B. is admitted from a long-term care facility with heart failure. As the physician examines the patient, she notes a pressure ulcer with necrotized tissue. The physician schedules the patient for _____ to remove the necrotized tissue from the wound.

10. A patient develops hives during a blood transfusion. The physician prescribes diphenhydramine, a(n) _____, to relieve the patient's itching.

Your name: _____

Competency Verification

Number of correct responses: _____ × 10 = _____ %

Clinical Connection Activity—Chapter 6: Digestive System

Objective: Apply your knowledge by selecting appropriate medical terms used in the clinical environment.

anorexia	hematemesis
antiemetic	intussusception
ascites	jaundice
colostomy	melena
dyspepsia	obstipation
emesis	peptic ulcer disease

Complete the statements by selecting a medical term from the list above.

1. A patient with a history of alcohol abuse tests positive for *Helicobacter pylori* bacteria. This bacterium places the patient at risk for _____.

2. Jane S., a 28-year-old patient with a history of IV drug abuse, is admitted with hepatitis. Her liver is no longer able to remove bilirubin, making her skin appear yellow. This condition is documented as _____.

3. A patient complains of nausea after undergoing a thoracotomy for treatment of lung cancer. The physician prescribes prochlorperazine, a(n) _____, to control his nausea and vomiting.

4. Sara G., a 15-month-old child, is brought to the emergency department by her mother because she has been crying inconsolably. An abdominal x-ray reveals _____, telescoping of the intestine within itself, which requires immediate surgical intervention.

5. A patient with a history of alcohol abuse arrives in the emergency department vomiting blood. This condition is documented as _____.

6. John G., a 59-year-old pharmacist, is diagnosed with colon cancer. His physician discusses treatment options and explains that he will most likely need a(n) _____, the creation of an opening of the colon through the abdominal wall.

7. During an admission assessment, a 79-year-old patient complains of indigestion after eating. This finding is documented as _____.

8. A 36-year-old patient with a history of alcohol abuse and cirrhosis of the liver has difficulty breathing. The patient has an abnormal accumulation of fluid in the abdomen, which is interfering with her breathing. This abnormal abdominal finding is known as _____.

9. Susan R., a 42-year-old teacher diagnosed with breast cancer, undergoes chemotherapy. After her first treatment she complains of _____, a term for appetite loss.

10. An 83-year-old patient with a history of arthritis comes to the emergency department complaining of weakness and fatigue. During the history, she reveals that her stool appears dark-colored and tarry. The physician documents this finding as _____.

Your name: _____

Competency Verification

Number of correct responses: _____ × 10 = _____ %

Clinical Connection Activity—Chapter 7: Respiratory System

Objective: Apply your knowledge by selecting appropriate medical terms used in the clinical environment.

acute respiratory distress syndrome	rale
influenza	sputum culture
Mantoux test	stridor
oximetry	tachypnea
pertussis	tracheostomy
polysomnography	tuberculosis

Complete the statements by selecting a medical term from the list above.

1. A patient comes to the emergency department complaining of fever, chills, headache, generalized muscle pain, and loss of appetite. The physician diagnoses _____, an acute infectious respiratory viral infection.

2. Yung L., a 47-year-old immigrant from Korea, comes to the emergency department complaining of a cough, weight loss, and night sweats. He is immediately placed on airborne isolation precautions because he is suspected of having a communicable disease that is spread by droplets contained in respiratory secretions. This disease is known as _____.

3. A patient diagnosed with pneumonia is admitted to the intensive care unit. Pulse _____ is used to assess the percentage of hemoglobin saturated with oxygen in the patient's blood.

4. James S., a 24-year-old bartender, is admitted to the hospital after sustaining severe chest trauma in a motor vehicle accident. His respiratory status deteriorates, requiring mechanical ventilation. On day two of his hospitalization, the patient's breathing worsens, and his lungs no longer function effectively, and the physician suspects _____.

5. An 84-year-old patient is admitted from a nursing home with pneumonia. The physician orders a(n) _____ to identify the causative organism so he can prescribe an effective antibiotic.

6. Noleen T. develops ventilator-dependent respiratory failure. During the second week of her hospitalization, the physician recommends a(n) _____, a surgical procedure in which an opening is made into the trachea to insert a breathing tube.

7. The nurse from the local middle school notifies parents that six students have become ill. These students were all diagnosed with _____, also known as whooping cough.

8. A patient with a history of heart failure arrives at the emergency department complaining of shortness of breath. Vital signs show that the patient's respiratory rate is 32 breaths/minute. A term for this finding is _____.

9. A 54-year-old patient admitted with upper gastrointestinal bleeding is prescribed two units of packed red blood cells. Five minutes after the blood transfusion begins, the patient's breathing becomes high-pitched and harsh. This finding is known as _____.

10. The infection control nurse reports that you have been inadvertently exposed to a patient with tuberculosis. You are instructed to report for a _____ to determine tuberculin sensitivity.

Your name: _____

Competency Verification

Number of correct responses: _____ × 10 = _____%

Clinical Connection Activity—Chapter 8: Cardiovascular System

beta blocker	ICD
bradycardia	mitral valve prolapse
CABG	pacemaker
cardioversion	statin
electrocardiogram	tachycardia
endocarditis	thrombectomy

Complete the statements by selecting a medical term from the list above.

1. Michael N. comes to the emergency department complaining of chest pain, nausea, and shortness of breath. The diagnostic test ordered for this patient is a(n) _____, a test that records electrical activity of his heart.

2. A patient arrives at the emergency department complaining of weakness and dizziness. The results of a cardiac monitor test show that the patient's heart rate is 36 beats/minute. This condition is known as _____.

3. A 75-year-old patient is brought to the emergency department after collapsing at the mall. The mall staff immediately used the automated external defibrillator (AED), which successfully converted the patient's heart rhythm. After a series of tests, the physician explains to the patient that he will require a(n) _____, a device that monitors and automatically corrects ventricular fibrillation.

4. Jennifer S. comes to the emergency department complaining of chest and left arm pain. The physician assesses the patient and immediately notifies the cardiac catheterization laboratory of the need for emergency catheterization. The catheterization shows that the patient needs an emergent _____, a surgical procedure that uses a vessel graft from another part of the body to circumvent a blocked portion of the coronary artery.

5. George F., a 36-year-old computer programmer, is diagnosed with hypertension. His physician prescribes, metoprolol, a(n) _____ to control his blood pressure.

6. A 55-year-old patient is admitted to the hospital with a pulseless, cool right leg. The surgeon examines the patient and explains that he will need a(n) _____ to remove the clot from his blood vessel.

7. After undergoing a lung biopsy, a patient develops an arrhythmia known as *atrial fibrillation*. The cardiologist recommends _____ to restore the patient's heart rhythm by applying a controlled electrical shock.

8. Jack H., a 62-year-old microbiologist, goes to his physician for a routine check-up. The blood tests that he had a week before his appointment show hypercholesterolemia. The physician prescribes simvastatin (Zocor), a(n) _____ to lower the patient's cholesterol.

9. Mary W. arrives at the emergency department with pain in her chest and shortness of breath. After performing various tests, the cardiologist notes that the bicuspid valve enters the left atrium during systole. This condition is known as _____.

10. After a 2-week stay in the intensive care unit, a patient develops methicillin-resistant *Staphylococcus aureus* bacteremia. The cardiologist orders an echocardiogram because bacteremia places the patient at risk for _____, an inflammation of the inner lining of the heart and its valves.

Your name: _____

Competency Verification

Number of correct responses: _____ × 10 = _____%

Clinical Connection Activity—Chapter 9: Blood, Lymph, and Immune Systems

Objective: **Apply your knowledge by selecting appropriate medical terms used in the clinical environment.**

AIDS	infectious mononucleosis
ALL	prothrombin time
AML	pruritus
autologous	septicemia
differential count	thrombolytic
edema	white blood cell count

Complete the statements by selecting a medical term from the list above.

1. A 22-year-old patient with a history of IV drug abuse arrives at the clinic complaining of fever, night sweats, and weight loss. The physician suspects _____, an infectious disease caused by the human immunodeficiency virus.

2. A patient is diagnosed with heart failure. During assessment, the patient's feet show an abnormal accumulation of fluid, a condition known as _____.

3. Brittany E., a college freshman, tells her roommate that she has a sore throat, tiredness, fever, and swollen neck glands. Brittany's roommate encourages her to go to the college infirmary, where the nurse suspects _____, an acute infection caused by the Epstein-Barr virus.

4. A 73-year-old patient is admitted from a long-term care facility with fever and chills. Blood cultures identify the presence of *Escherichia coli*. The physician diagnoses _____, also known as a blood infection.

5. Kate S. is brought to the emergency department by her husband because she has had a fever for the past 3 days. Blood specimens are drawn and her white blood cell count is elevated. The physician asks the laboratory staff to perform a(n) _____ to determine the distribution of white blood cells.

6. A 66-year-old patient admitted with uncontrolled atrial fibrillation is started on the anticoagulant warfarin (Coumadin). The physician orders a(n) _____ to monitor the effectiveness of warfarin therapy.

7. A week before undergoing back surgery, Jamal S. donated his own blood for use during surgery. A transfusion prepared from the patient's blood is known as a(n) _____ transfusion.

8. Beth A. is diagnosed with Hodgkin lymphoma. Her presenting symptoms included lymph node enlargement in the left side of the neck, weight loss, fever, and extreme itching, also known as _____.

9. A patient arrives at the emergency department complaining of substernal chest pain. The electrocardiogram (ECG) and other tests identify a clot in the coronary artery. The cardiologist prescribes alteplase (Activase), a _____ to treat this condition.

10. After undergoing a bone marrow biopsy, Ricardo M. is diagnosed with acute myelogenous leukemia. The physician might abbreviate this diagnosis as _____.

Your name: _____

Competency Verification

Number of correct responses: _____ × 10 = _____%

Clinical Connection Activity—Chapter 10: Musculoskeletal System

Objective: Apply your knowledge by selecting appropriate medical terms used in the clinical environment.

arthritis	dorsiflexion
ACL	femur
AK	laminectomy
arthroscopy	NSAID
bone density test	skeletal muscle relaxant
crepitation	total hip replacement

Complete the statements by selecting a medical term from the list above.

1. Jimmy R., a 26-year-old minor league baseball player sustains an ankle injury. The athletic trainer assesses the patient's ankle by elevating his foot. This motion is known as _____.

2. A 19-year-old unrestrained driver is brought to the emergency department after sustaining injuries in a motor vehicle accident. The patient complains of pain in his left thigh. An x-ray reveals a fracture of the thigh bone, called the _____.

3. Evelyn K., a 56-year-old patient comes to the clinic complaining of pain in her knees. The nurse practitioner assesses the patient and suspects _____, an inflammation of the joints.

4. Tim B., a high school senior, sustains a knee injury in a high school football game. Knee x-rays reveal a torn ligament. The orthopedic surgeon recommends _____, a procedure in which a small surgical instrument is inserted into the joint to repair the ligament.

5. Wayne D., a 52-year-old salesman, is referred to the orthopedic surgeon for treatment of a herniated disk. The surgeon tells the patient that he must undergo a(n) _____ to remove the herniated disk.

6. While assessing a 56-year-old patient with right shoulder pain, you note a dry grating sound as she moves her arm. You document this finding as _____.

7. A 42-year-old tennis player is diagnosed with tendinitis of the right elbow. The physician prescribes ibuprofen (Motrin), a(n) _____, to treat the acute musculoskeletal condition.

8. A 52-year-old patient goes to the family practice physician for a routine examination. The physician recommends a(n) _____ to determine whether demineralization from osteoporosis has occurred.

9. A basketball player arrives at the emergency department after sustaining an anterior cruciate ligament injury. The physician might abbreviate this as an injury of the _____.

10. John G., a hospital maintenance worker, injures his back while working. The employee health physician prescribes methocarbamol and aspirin (Flexeril), a(n) _____, to relieve his muscle spasms.

Your name: _____

Competency Verification

Number of correct responses: _____ × 10 = _____%

Clinical Connection Activity—Chapter 11: Genitourinary System

Objective: **Apply your knowledge by selecting appropriate medical terms used in the clinical environment.**

bacteriuria	hydronephrosis
calculus	nocturia
dialysis	oliguria
diuretic	PSA
electrolyte	TURP
hematuria	vasectomy

Complete the statements by selecting a medical term from the list above.

1. Three days after being admitted to the intensive care unit, Jennifer S. develops a fever and elevated white blood cell count. A urine culture performed on this patient is positive for bacteria. This condition is known as _____.

2. An indwelling urinary catheter is placed in a patient admitted with fever and hypotension. Her urine specimen reveals red blood cells. This finding is documented as _____.

3. A patient with end-stage renal disease comes to the nephrologist's office for a routine examination. The patient's laboratory test results show a serious elevation of nitrogenous wastes in the blood, requiring _____, a procedure that filters these wastes from the bloodstream.

4. James J. comes to the urologist's office for consultation. After the birth of their third child, James and his wife decide that he should undergo a _____, a method of male contraception in which the vas deferens is excised.

5. A 54-year-old man arrives at the emergency department with urinary retention. The physician examines him and diagnoses benign prostatic hyperplasia. The next morning, the patient undergoes _____, a surgical procedure that uses a resectoscope to chip away at the prostate.

6. Srijana P. is admitted to the coronary care unit with heart failure. The cardiologist prescribes furosemide (Lasix), a(n) _____, to increase her excretion of urine.

7. Donovan M., a 32-year-old computer programmer, arrives at the outpatient dialysis center for his first treatment. A blood specimen is obtained to evaluate _____ levels, which include potassium, sodium, and calcium.

8. A 45-year-old patient arrives at the physician's office complaining of frequent urination at night. The physician documents this finding as _____.

9. The physician orders a(n) _____ as part of a patient's annual examination. This test is used to detect prostate cancer.

10. Brenda L. develops severe left flank pain while attending her friend's wedding. Her husband brings her to the emergency department where she is diagnosed with a kidney stone. The clinical term for kidney stone is _____.

Your name: _____

Competency Verification

Number of correct responses: _____ × 10 = _____ %

Clinical Connection Activity—Chapter 12: Female Reproductive System

Objective: Apply your knowledge by selecting appropriate medical terms used in the clinical environment.

abruptio placentae
breech presentation
cephalopelvic disproportion
chlamydia
conization
dysmenorrhea

ectopic pregnancy
FHT
FSH
hysterectomy
lumpectomy
oral contraceptives

Complete the statements by selecting a medical term from the list above.

1. Julia S., a 17-year-old high school student, complains of severe pain with menstruation. Her complaint is documented as _____.

2. A group of junior high school students is studying sexually transmitted diseases (STDs). They learn that _____ is the most prevalent and one of the most damaging STDs in the United States.

3. A 16-year-old arrives at the clinic for birth control counseling. After weighing her options, she decides that birth control pills, also know as _____, are her best option because they are highly reliable and easy to use.

4. During her 30th week of pregnancy, Joan G. experiences vaginal bleeding. The obstetrician diagnoses _____, the premature separation of the placenta.

5. Keisha M. has an ultrasound during her 36th week of pregnancy, which reveals that the feet of the fetus are presenting first. On the ultrasound report, the radiologist documents this finding as _____.

6. Ellen S. comes to the emergency department complaining of abdominal pain. Computed tomography of the abdomen reveals a(n) _____, a condition in which an ovum has implanted in the fallopian tube.

7. The gynecologist calls Judy S. to inform her that her Papanicolaou test result is abnormal. He recommends that she return for _____, an excision of a cone-shaped piece of cervical tissue for histological examination.

8. The obstetrician writes in the patient's progress note that he suspects CPD in a patient who is 38 weeks pregnant. This finding indicates a(n) _____.

9. Rosalie W. arrives at the hospital in active labor. You assess fetal heart tones and document your findings in the medical record. You might use _____ to abbreviate fetal heart tones.

10. Susan H., a 36-year-old mother of twins, finds a lump in her left breast while performing breast self-examination. After mammography shows a small tumor, the physician recommends a(n) _____, excision of the breast tumor.

Your name: _____

Competency Verification

Number of correct responses: _____ × 10 = _____%

Clinical Connection Activity—Chapter 13: Endocrine System

Objective: **Apply your knowledge by selecting appropriate medical terms used in the clinical environment.**

antidiuretic	hyponatremia
corticosteroid	MRI
diabetic ketoacidosis	oral antidiabetic
gestational diabetes	polyphagia
hyperkalemia	radioactive iodine uptake
hypoglycemia	thyroid scan

Complete the statements by selecting a medical term from the list above.

1. A type 2 diabetic patient becomes diaphoretic and pale and complains of feeling shaky 30 minutes after administration of insulin. The probable cause is _____, an abnormally low glucose level.

2. Bernadette D. develops diabetes during her second trimester of pregnancy. This condition is known as _____.

3. Franklin Z., a 19-year-old college student with a history of type 1 diabetes, arrives at the emergency department complaining of nausea, vomiting, and urinary frequency. Routine laboratory test results reveal a severely elevated blood glucose level. His admitting diagnosis is DKA, which is an abbreviation that means _____.

4. A patient with a history of end-stage renal disease is brought to the emergency department by his wife. He is drowsy and his heartbeat is irregular. Routine blood studies show an elevated potassium level. This finding is known as _____.

5. Sharon C. arrives at the physician's office because she has been experiencing weight gain. When the physician examines her neck, he notes an enlargement. The physician orders a(n) _____ to determine the cause of swelling in the neck.

6. Joya B. is brought to the emergency department after suffering a seizure at work. Routine laboratory studies show a low sodium level, which is documented as _____.

7. During a seminar nursing students are learning the signs and symptoms of diabetes, which include polydipsia, polyuria, and _____.

8. Ivan R., a 63-year-old police department dispatcher with a 40-year history of smoking, is admitted with abdominal pain and weight loss. The physician suspects pancreatic cancer and orders a(n) _____, an imaging technique that uses radio waves and a strong magnetic field to aid the diagnosis.

9. Stan T., a 17-year-old high school student, develops diabetes insipidus after sustaining a head injury in a motor vehicle accident. The physician prescribes vasopressin (Pitressin), a(n) _____, to reduce the patient's urine output.

10. Dale B., a 64-year-old security consultant, is diagnosed with type 2 diabetes. His physician prescribes glipizide (Glucotrol), a(n) _____, to stimulate the pancreas to increase insulin production and decrease peripheral insulin resistance.

Your name: _____

Competency Verification

Number of correct responses: _____ × 10 = _____ %

Clinical Connection Activity—Chapter 14: Nervous System

Objective: Apply your knowledge by selecting appropriate medical terms used in the clinical environment.

aphasia	PET scan
concussion	psychostimulant
hemiparesis	Reye syndrome
hydrocephalus	spinal tap
hypnotic	stroke
meninges	TIA

Complete the statements by selecting a medical term from the list above.

1. An 18-year-old college freshman arrives at the college infirmary complaining of a headache, body aches, and fever. The nurse sends the student to the emergency department because she suspects meningitis, an infection involving the
_____.

2. The emergency medical technician alerts the emergency department that they are en route with a patient who is experiencing
_____, paralysis on the right side. The emergency department nurse alerts the stroke team so they can intervene immediately when the patient arrives in the emergency department.

3. Katherine W., an 82-year-old nursing home resident, is brought to the emergency department with difficulty speaking and facial droop. The physician suspects a(n) _____, also known as a cerebrovascular accident.

4. Jennifer S., a 64-year-old teacher, suddenly develops difficulty speaking and dizziness. By the time she reaches the emergency department, her symptoms abate. The physician suspects that the patient experienced a temporary interference with the blood supply to the brain, known as a
_____.

5. Rachael M., a 21-year-old college student, arrives at the emergency department complaining of headache, fever, and neck stiffness. The neurologist

suspects meningitis, so he performs a lumbar puncture, also known as a _____, to confirm the diagnosis.

6. A 14-year-old junior high school student is brought to the emergency department after having a seizure in the school library. To determine whether the patient has epilepsy, the physician orders a(n) _____ to record the metabolic activity in brain tissue.

7. On admission, Luella W., a stroke patient, was unable to speak. The nurse documented this condition as _____.

8. Kyra N. is admitted to the intensive care unit after sustaining a closed head injury in a motor vehicle accident. Forty-eight hours after the injury, the patient is confused and agitated. The neurosurgeon orders a CT scan of the head. The CT scan shows _____, an accumulation of fluid in the ventricles in the brain, causing increased intracranial pressure.

9. An 11-year-old child with influenza symptoms is brought to the pediatrician's office by his mother. The pediatrician advises the mother to give her child plenty of fluids and acetaminophen (Tylenol) for fever, as needed. Acetaminophen is recommended to control fever because aspirin is associated with _____ in children with acute viral infection.

10. Trent F., a 6-year-old patient, is diagnosed with attention deficit hyperactivity disorder. The pediatrician prescribes methylphenidate (Ritalin), a(n)
_____.

Your name: _____

Competency Verification

Number of correct responses: _____ × 10 = _____ %

Clinical Connection Activity—Chapter 15: Special Senses: Eyes and Ears

Objective: **Apply your knowledge by selecting appropriate medical terms used in the clinical environment.**

antiemetic	IOP
antiglaucoma agent	otitis media
cochlear implant	photophobia
dacryocystography	tinnitus
exophthalmos	tympanoplasty
IOL	wax emulsifier

Complete the statements by selecting a medical term from the list above.

1. A 2-year-old child with a 5-day history of an upper respiratory tract infection is brought to the pediatrician's office by her mother. The mother states that her child has been irritable and pulling at her ears. The pediatrician examines the child's ears and diagnoses _____, inflammation of the middle ear.

2. Eileen A., a 32-year-old designer, is diagnosed with a hyperactive thyroid. One of her presenting symptoms is the protrusion of both eyeballs, known as _____.

3. A patient diagnosed with viral meningitis complains of an unusual intolerance and sensitivity to light. You document this finding as _____.

4. Ruth T., an 88-year-old patient with osteoarthritis, arrives at the physician's office complaining of ringing in her ears. The patient explains that she has been taking aspirin for her arthritis. The physician explains that she is suffering from _____, an adverse effect of high-dose aspirin therapy.

5. A patient comes to the ophthalmologist's office complaining of excess tearing. The ophthalmologist orders _____, a radiographic imaging of the nasolacrimal glands and ducts to determine the cause.

6. Juan C. is referred to the otolaryngologist because of hearing loss. The otolaryngologist recommends a(n) _____, an artificial hearing device that produces hearing sensations by stimulating nerves within the inner ear.

7. Gary D., a second-grade student with a history of frequent ear infections, is diagnosed with hearing loss and referred to the otolaryngologist. The tolaryngologist examines the child and discovers a perforation in the left eardrum. Reconstruction of the eardrum, a procedure known as _____, is scheduled.

8. A 67-year-old grocery store clerk is diagnosed with glaucoma. Timolol (Betimol), a(n) _____, is prescribed to decrease aqueous humor production in the patient's eyes.

9. Kathleen J., a 42-year-old homemaker, is brought to the physician's office by her husband. She has been suffering from vertigo, nausea, and vomiting for the past 3 days. The physician prescribes meclizine (Antrizine), a(n) _____, to combat the patient's symptoms.

10. The ophthalmologist discovers that a patient has increased intraocular pressure. You might abbreviate this finding as increased _____.

Your name: _____

Competency Verification

Number of correct responses: _____ × 10 = _____ %

CLINICAL CONNECTION ACTIVITY ANSWER KEY

Chapter 5: Integumentary System

1. parasiticide
2. alopecia
3. metastasis
4. eschar
5. cellulitis
6. petechiae
7. scabies
8. tuberculosis
9. debridement
10. antihistamine

Chapter 6: Digestive System

1. peptic ulcer disease
2. jaundice
3. antiemetic
4. intussusception
5. hematemesis
6. colostomy
7. dyspepsia
8. ascites
9. anorexia
10. melena

Chapter 7: Respiratory System

1. influenza
2. tuberculosis
3. oximetry
4. ARDS
5. sputum culture
6. tracheostomy
7. pertussis
8. tachypnea
9. stridor
10. Mantoux test

Chapter 8: Cardiovascular System

1. electrocardiogram
2. bradycardia
3. ICD
4. CABG
5. beta blocker
6. thrombectomy
7. cardioversion
8. statin
9. mitral valve prolapse
10. endocarditis

Chapter 9: Blood, Lymph, and Immune Systems

1. AIDS
2. edema
3. infectious mononucleosis
4. septicemia
5. differential count
6. prothrombin time
7. autologous
8. pruritus
9. thrombolytic
10. AML

Chapter 10: Musculoskeletal System

1. dorsiflexion
2. femur
3. arthritis
4. arthroscopy
5. laminectomy
6. crepitation
7. NSAID
8. bone density test
9. ACL
10. muscle relaxant

Chapter 11: Genitourinary System

1. bacteriuria
2. hematuria
3. dialysis
4. vasectomy
5. TURP
6. diuretic
7. electrolyte
8. nocturia
9. PSA
10. calculus

Chapter 12: Female Reproductive System

1. dysmenorrhea
2. chlamydia
3. oral contraceptive pills
4. abruptio placentae
5. breech presentation
6. ectopic pregnancy
7. conization
8. cephalopelvic disproportion
9. FHT
10. lumpectomy

Chapter 13: Endocrine System

1. hypoglycemia
2. gestational diabetes
3. diabetic ketoacidosis
4. hyperkalemia
5. thyroid scan
6. hyponatremia
7. polyphagia
8. MRI
9. antidiuretic
10. oral antidiabetic

Chapter 14: Nervous System

1. meninges
2. hemiparesis
3. stroke
4. TIA
5. spinal tap
6. PET scan
7. aphasia
8. hydrocephalus
9. Reye syndrome
10. psychostimulant

Chapter 15: Special Senses: Eyes and Ears

1. otitis media
2. exophthalmos
3. photophobia
4. tinnitus
5. dacryocystography
6. cochlear implant
7. tympanoplasty
8. antiglaucoma agent
9. antiemetic
10. IOP

Flowchart Activity—Chapter 6: Digestive System

Objective: Apply your knowledge of anatomy and physiology by completing the flowchart for the physiological processes listed below.

The digestive system, also called the *gastrointestinal tract,* forms a tube that begins at the mouth, where food enters the body. It terminates at the anus, where solid waste substances are eliminated from the body. Follow the digestive process by listing, in order, the pathway of structures (listed below) involved in digestion. The first structure is listed for you.

anus
ascending colon
cecum
descending colon
duodenum

esophagus
ileum
jejunum
pharynx (throat)
rectum

sigmoid colon
stomach
transverse colon

Pathway of Food Through The Digestive System

mouth _____

↓ _____

↓ _____

↓ _____

↓ _____

↓ _____

↓ _____

↓ _____

↓ _____

↓ _____

↓ _____

↓ _____

↓ _____

↓ _____

Feces are expelled _____

Flowchart Activity—Chapter 7: Respiratory System

Objective: **Apply your knowledge of anatomy and physiology by completing the flowchart for the physiological processes listed below.**
Air is drawn into the nasal cavity, where it is filtered, heated, and moistened to prepare for its journey to the lungs. Follow the pathway of inhaled air from the nose to the lung capillaries by listing, in order, the structures (listed below) through which air passes. The first structure is listed for you.

alveoli
bronchi
bronchioles
larynx (voice box)

lung capillaries
nasal cavities
pharynx (throat)
trachea

Pathway of Inhaled Air (Oxygenated) in the Respiratory System

nose (nares)
↓

↓

↓

↓

↓

↓

↓

(bloodstream)

Flowchart Activity—Chapter 8: Cardiovascular System

Objective: Apply your knowledge of anatomy and physiology by completing the flowchart for the physiological processes listed below.

The cardiovascular system is composed of the heart and blood vessels. As the heart pumps blood, vast numbers of intricate blood vessels deliver the blood to all cells of the body. Follow the pathway of oxygen-poor blood as it enters the heart, converts to oxygen-rich blood, and travels to all parts of the body by listing, in order, the structures (listed below) through which the blood flows.

aorta	lungs	right atrium
left atrium	pulmonary arteries	right ventricle
left ventricle	pulmonary veins	venae cavae

Pathway of Blood as It Enters and Leaves the Heart

Oxygen-poor blood flows from all parts of the body.
↓

_____

Systemic circulation

_____
↓

Heart

_____
↓
tricuspid valve
↓

_____
↓
pulmonary semilunar valve
↓

Pulmonary circulation
↓

_____
↓

_____
↓

_____

↓

Heart
↓
_____
↓
bicuspid valve
↓
_____
↓
aortic semilunar valve
↓

Systemic circulation
↓
_____
↓
Oxygen-rich blood flows to all parts of the body.

Flowchart Activity—Chapter 11: Genitourinary System

The primary purpose of the urinary system is to help maintain a constant balance (homeostasis) of water, salts, and acids in body fluids and removes waste products from the blood by excreting them in the urine. Follow the urinary process of forming and excreting urine from the body by completing the following flow chart. The first structure is listed for you.

bladder
kidney
meatus
nephron

renal pelvis
ureter
urethra

Pathway of Urine Formation and Excretion Through the Urinary System

renal artery
↓
_____
↓
_____
↓
_____
↓
_____
↓
_____
↓
_____
↓
_____

ANSWER KEY FOR FLOWCHART ACTIVITIES

Chapter 6: Digestive System

mouth
↓
pharynx
↓
esophagus
↓
stomach
↓
duodenum
↓
jejunum
↓
ileum
↓
cecum
↓
ascending colon
↓
transverse colon
↓
descending colon
↓
sigmoid colon
↓
rectum
↓
anus

Chapter 7: Respiratory System

nose (nares)
↓
nasal cavities
↓
pharynx (throat)
↓
larynx (voice box)
↓
trachea
↓
bronchi
↓
bronchioles
↓
alveoli
↓
lung capillaries (bloodstream)

Chapter 8: Cardiovascular System

Oxygen-poor blood flows from all parts of the body.
↓

Systemic circulation

venae cavae
↓

Heart

right atrium
↓
tricuspid valve
↓
right ventricle
↓
pulmonary semilunar valve
↓

Pulmonary circulation

↓
pulmonary arteries
↓
lungs
↓
pulmonary veins
↓

Heart

↓
left atrium
↓
bicuspid valve
↓
left ventricle
↓
aortic semilunar valve
↓

Systemic circulation

↓
aorta
↓
Oxygen-rich blood flows to all parts of the body.

Chapter 11: Genitourinary System

renal artery
↓
kidney
↓
nephron
↓
renal pelvis
↓
ureter
↓
bladder
↓
urethra
↓
meatus

Pronunciation and Spelling Activity— Chapter 5: Integumentary System

Objective: To correctly spell and pronounce the medical terms in the table below

Pronunciation Instructions

1. Cover the Pronunciation Key column with a sheet of paper and say each word aloud.
2. Uncover the Pronunciation Key column and check whether you have said the word correctly.
3. Place a check (✓) mark in the column if you pronounced the word correctly.

Spelling Instructions

1. Have a peer dictate each medical term below using the Pronunciation Key column as a guide.
2. As each word is dictated, write it on a separate paper or enter it into a word-processing document.
3. Correct your spelling using the list below.
4. Place a Check (✓) mark in the column if you pronounced the medical word correctly. Your instructor will then select 10 words for you to pronounce as a quiz.

Pronunciation Key	Medical Term	Pronounced Correctly ✓	Spelled Correctly ✓
ĂK-nē	acne		
ā-TĬP-ĭ-kăl	atypical		
KĂR-bŭng-kĕl	carbuncle		
dā-brēd-MŎN	debridement		
dĕr-mă-TŎL-ō-jĭst	dermatologist		
ĕr-ĭ-THĒ-mă	erythema		
ĔS-kăr	eschar		
FŪ-rŭng-k'l	furuncle		
hō-mē-ō-STĀ-sĭs	homeostasis		
hī-drō-KOR-tĭ-sōn	hydrocortisone		
hī-pĕr-kĕr-ă-TŌ-sĭs	hyperkeratosis		
LĪ-dō-kān	lidocaine		
pē-TĒ-kē-ă	petechia		
pī-lō-NĪ-dăl	pilonidal		
sō-RĪ-ă-sĭs	psoriasis		
SKĀ-bēz	scabies		
sŭb-kū-TĀ-nē-ŭs	subcutaneous		

Pronunciation Key	Medical Term	Pronounced Correctly ✓	Spelled Correctly ✓
TĬN-ē-ăh	tinea		
ŭr-tĭ-KĀ-rē-ă	urticaria		
vĭt-ĭl-Ī-gō	vitiligo		

Your name: _____

Competency Verification

Number of correct pronunciations: _____ × 10
= _____ %
Number of correct spellings: _____ × 10
= _____ %

Pronunciation and Spelling Activity— Chapter 6: Digestive System

Objective: To correctly spell and pronounce the medical terms in the table below

Pronunciation Instructions

1. Cover the Pronunciation Key column with a sheet of paper and say each word aloud.
2. Uncover the Pronunciation Key column and check whether you have said the word correctly.
3. Place a check (✓) mark in the column if you pronounced the word correctly.

Spelling Instructions

1. Have a peer dictate each medical term below using the Pronunciation Key column as a guide.
2. As each word is dictated, write it on a separate paper or enter it into a word-processing document.
3. Correct your spelling using the list below.
4. Place a check (✓) mark in the column if you pronounced the medical word correctly. Your instructor will then pick 10 words for you to pronounce as a quiz.

Pronunciation Key	Medical Term	Pronounced Correctly ✓	Spelled Correctly ✓
ĕr-ō-FĀ-jē-ă	aerophagia		
ă-năs-tō-MŌ-sĭs	anastomosis		
ă-SĪ-tēz	ascites		
ā-sĭmp-tō-MĂT-ĭk	asymptomatic		
kă-KĔKS-ē-ă	cachexia		
KĪ-lō-plăs-tē	cheiloplasty		
kō-lē-sĭs-TŎG-ră-fē	cholecystography		
kō-lē-lĭ-THĪ-ă-sĭs	cholelithiasis		
sĭr-RŌ-sĭs	cirrhosis		
kō-LŎS-tō-mē	colostomy		
ĔKS-ō-krĭn	exocrine		
găs-TRĂL-jē-ă	gastralgia		
ĭl-ē-ŎS-tō-mē	ileostomy		
SĬL-ē-ŭm	psyllium		
pī-lō-rō-mī-ŎT-ō-mē	pyloromyotomy		
rē-gŭr-jĭ-TĀ-shŭn	regurgitation		
SFĬNGK-tĕr	sphincter		
stē-ă-tō-RĒ-ă	steatorrhea		
sŭb-LĬNG-gwăl	sublingual		
VĂR-ĭ-sēz	varices		

Your name: _____

Competency Verification

Number of correct pronunciations: _____ × 10
= _____ %
Number of correct spellings: _____ × 10
= _____ %

Pronunciation and Spelling Activity—Chapter 7: Respiratory System

Objective: To correctly spell and pronounce the medical terms in the table below

Pronunciation Instructions

1. Cover the Pronunciation Key column with a sheet of paper and say each word aloud.
2. Uncover the Pronunciation Key column and check whether you have said the word correctly.
3. Place a check (✓) mark in the column if you pronounced the word correctly.

Spelling Instructions

1. Have a peer dictate each medical term below using the Pronunciation Key column as a guide.
2. As each word is dictated, write it on a separate paper or enter it into a word-processing document.
3. Correct your spelling using the list below.
4. Place a check (✓) mark in the column if you pronounced the medical word correctly. Your instructor will then select 10 words for you to pronounce as a quiz.

Pronunciation Key	Medical Term	Pronounced Correctly ✓	Spelled Correctly ✓
ăs-ĭ-DŌ-sĭs	acidosis		
ĂR-ō-sŏl	aerosol		
ăl-BŪ-tĕr-ăl	albuterol		
ăn-ŎZ-mē-ă	anosmia		
brŏng-KŎS-kō-pē	bronchoscopy		
KŌ-dēn	codeine		
dĭsp-NĒ-ă	dyspnea		
hē-MŎP-tĭ-sĭs	hemoptysis		
lăr-ĭn-GŎS-kō-pē	laryngoscopy		
lă-VĂZH	lavage		
mē-dē-ăs-tĭ-NŎS-kō-pē	mediastinoscopy		
ŏk-SĬM-ă-trē	oximetry		
ploor-ĔK-tō-mē	pleurectomy		
nū-mō-kō-nē-Ō-sĭs	pneumoconiosis		
pī-ō-THŌ-răks	pyothorax		
RĪ-nō-plăs-tē	rhinoplasty		
RŎNG-kŭs	rhonchus		
sĕp-tō-PLĂS-tē	septoplasty		
spī-RŎM-ĕ-trē	spirometry		
thō-ră-sĕn-TĒ-sĭs	thoracentesis		

Your name: _____

Competency Verification

Number of correct pronunciations: _____ × 10
= _____ %
Number of correct spellings: _____ × 10
= _____ %

Pronunciation and Spelling Activity— Chapter 8: Cardiovascular System

Objective: To correctly spell and pronounce the medical terms in the list below

Pronunciation Instructions

1. Cover the Pronunciation Key column with a sheet of paper and say each word aloud.
2. Uncover the Pronunciation Key column and check whether you have said the word correctly.
3. Place a check (✓) mark in the column if you pronounced the word correctly.

Spelling instructions

1. Have a peer dictate each medical term below using the Pronunciation Key column as a guide.
2. As each word is dictated, write it on a separate paper or enter it into a word-processing document.
3. Correct your spelling using the list below.
4. Place a check (✓) mark in the column if you pronounced the medical word correctly. Your instructor will then select 10 words for you to pronounce as a quiz.

Pronunciation Key	Medical Term	Pronounced Correctly ✓	Spelled Correctly ✓
ĂN-jē-ō-plăs-tē	angioplasty		
ā-or-TŎG-ră-fē	aortography		
ă-RĬTH-mē-ă	arrhythmia		
ăr-tēr-ē-ō-LĪ-tĭs	arteriolitis		
ăr-tē-rē-ō-sklĕ-RŌ-sĭs	arteriosclerosis		
KĂR-dē-ō-vĕr-zhŭn	cardioversion		
kăth-ĕ-tĕr-ĭ-ZĀ-shŭn	catheterization		
kō-ărk-TĀ-shŭn	coarctation		
kŏm-ĭ-shŭr-ŎT-ō-mē	commissurotomy		
ĕm-bō-lĭ-ZĀ-shŭn	embolization		
hī-pĕr-lĭp-ĭ-DĒ-mē-ă	hyperlipidemia		
ĭs-KĒ-mē-ă	ischemia		
mă-LĀZ	malaise		
nī-trō-GLĬS-ĕr-ĭn	nitroglycerin		
ŏ-KLOO-zhŭn	occlusion		
pĕr-FŪ-zhŭn	perfusion		
fō-nō-kăr-dē-ŎG-ră-fē	phonocardiography		
prō-fĭ-LĂK-sĭs	prophylaxis		
SFĬG-moyd	sphygmoid		
vĭs-KŎS-ĭ-tē	viscosity		

Your name: _____

Competency Verification

Number of correct pronunciations: _____ × 10
= _____ %
Number of correct spellings: _____ × 10
= _____ %

Pronunciation and Spelling Activity—Chapter 9: Blood, Lymph, and Immune Systems

Objective: To correctly spell and pronounce the medical terms in the table below

Pronunciation instructions

1. Cover the Pronunciation Key column with a sheet of paper and say each word aloud.
2. Uncover the Pronunciation Key column and check whether you have said the word correctly.
3. Place a Check (✓) mark in the column if you pronounced the word correctly.

Spelling instructions

1. Have a peer dictate each medical term below using the Pronunciation Key column as a guide.
2. As each word is dictated, write it on a separate paper or enter it into a word-processing document.
3. Correct your spelling using the list below.
4. Place a check (✓) mark in the column if you pronounced the medical word correctly. Your instructor will then select 10 words for you to pronounce as a quiz.

Pronunciation Key	Medical Term	Pronounced Correctly ✓	Spelled Correctly ✓
ĂL-ō-grăft	allograft		
ăs-pǐ-RĀ-shŭn	aspiration		
aw-TŎL-ō-gŭs	autologous		
ĕ-rǐth-rō-blăs-TŌ-sǐs	erythroblastosis		
hē-mō-glō-bǐ-NŎP-ă-thē	hemoglobinopathy		
hē-MŎL-ǐ-sǐs	hemolysis		
hē-mō-FŌ-bē-ă	hemophobia		
hē-mō-STĀ-sǐs	hemostasis		
HĚP-ă-rǐn	heparin		
ǐm-ū-nō-pă-THŎL-ō-jē	immunopathology		
ī-sō-KRŌM-ǐk	isochromic		
kăr-ē-ŎL-ǐ-sǐs	karyolysis		
LĬM-foyd	lymphoid		
lǐm-fō-săr-KŌ-mă	lymphosarcoma		
mŏn-ō-NŪ-klē-ăr	mononuclear		
mī-ĕ-lō-JĚN-ǐk	myelogenic		
PĂL-ē-ă-tǐv	palliative		
poy-kǐl-ō-sī-TŌ-sǐs	poikilocytosis		
sĕp-tǐ-SĒ-mē-ă	septicemia		
strĕp-tō-KĪ-nās	streptokinase		

Your name: _____

Competency Verification

Number of correct pronunciations: _____ × 10
= _____ %
Number of correct spellings: _____ × 10
= _____ %

Pronunciation and Spelling Activity— Chapter 10: Musculoskeletal System

Objective: **To correctly spell and pronounce the medical terms in the table below**

Pronunciation Instructions

1. Cover the Pronunciation Key column with a sheet of paper and say each word aloud.
2. Uncover the Pronunciation Key column and check whether you have said the word correctly.
3. Place a check (✓) mark in the column if you pronounced the word correctly.

Spelling Instructions

1. Have a peer dictate each medical term below using the Pronunciation Key column as a guide.
2. As each word is dictated, write it on a separate paper or enter it into a word-processing document.
3. Correct your spelling using the list below.
4. Place a check (✓) mark in the column if you pronounced the medical word correctly. Your instructor will then select 10 words for you to pronounce as a quiz.

Pronunciation Key	Medical Term	Pronounced Correctly ✓	Spelled Correctly ✓
ăng-kĭ-LŌ-sĭs	ankylosis		
ăr-THRĪ-tĭs	arthritis		
kăl-kăn-nē-ō-DĬN-ē-ă	calcaneodynia		
KĂL-sē-ŭm KĂR-bŏn-āt	calcium carbonate		
klăw-dĭ-KĀ-shŭn	claudication		
KROO-shē-āt	cruciate		
ē-lĕk-trō-mī-ŎG-ră-fē	electromyography		
hĕm-ă-tō-poy-Ē-sĭs	hematopoiesis		
ī-bū-PRŌ-fĕn	ibuprofen		
kī-FŌ-sĭs	kyphosis		
mĕt-ă-tăr-SĂL-jē-ă	metatarsalgia		
or-thō-PĒ-dĭst	orthopedist		
pē-dē-ĂT-rĭk	pediatric		
făl-ăn-JĔK-tō-mē	phalangectomy		
pō-DĪ-ă-trē	podiatry		
PRŎS-thē-sĭs	prosthesis		
spŏn-dĭ-LĪ-tĭs	spondylitis		
spŏn-dĭ-lō-lĭs-THĒ-sĭs	spondylolisthesis		
sŭb-lŭk-SĀ-shŭn	subluxation		
TĂL-ĭ-pēz	talipes		

Your name: _____

Competency Verification

Number of correct pronunciations: _____ × 10
= _____ %
Number of correct spellings: _____ × 10
= _____ %

Pronunciation and Spelling Activity—Chapter 11: Genitourinary System

Objective: To correctly spell and pronounce the medical terms in the table below

Pronunciation Instructions

1. Cover the Pronunciation Key column with a sheet of paper and say each word aloud.
2. Uncover the Pronunciation Key column and check whether you have said the word correctly.
3. Place a check (✓) mark in the column if you pronounced the word correctly.

Spelling instructions

1. Have a peer dictate each medical term below using the Pronunciation Key column as a guide.
2. As each word is dictated, write it on a separate paper or enter it into a word-processing document.
3. Correct your spelling using the list below.
4. Place a check (✓) mark in the column if you pronounced the medical word correctly. Your instructor will then select 10 words for you to pronounce as a quiz.

Pronunciation Key	Medical Term	Pronounced Correctly ✓	Spelled Correctly ✓
ăn-OR-kĭ-dĭzm	anorchidism		
ăz-ō-TĒ-mē-ă	azotemia		
băl-ă-NĪ-tĭs	balanitis		
krĭpt-OR-kĭd-ĭzm	cryptorchidism		
SĬST-ō-skōp	cystoscope		
dĭs-Ū-rē-ă	dysuria		
ĕn-ū-RĒ-sĭs	enuresis		
hī-pō-kă-LĒ-mē-ă	hypokalemia		
hī-pō-SPĀ-dē-ăs	hypospadias		
mē-ă-TŎT-ō-mē	meatotomy		
pĕr-kū-TĀ-nē-ŭs	percutaneous		
fī-MŌ-sĭs	phimosis		
PĪ-ĕ-lō-plăs-tē	pyeloplasty		
RĒ-flŭks	reflux		
tĕs-TŎS-tĕr-ōn	testosterone		
ū-rē-tĕr-ĔK-tă-sĭs	ureterectasis		
ū-rĭ-NĂL-ĭ-sĭs	urinalysis		
ū-rō-lĭ-THĪ-ă-sĭs	urolithiasis		
VĂR-ĭ-kō-sēl	varicocele		
văs-ō-PRĔS-ĭn	vasopressin		

Your name: _____

Competency Verification

Number of correct pronunciations: _____ $\times$ 10
= _____ %
Number of correct spellings: _____ $\times$ 10
= _____ %

Pronunciation and Spelling Activity—Chapter 12: Female Reproductive System

Objective: To correctly spell and pronounce the medical terms in the table below

Pronunciation instructions

1. Cover the Pronunciation Key column with a sheet of paper and say each word aloud.
2. Uncover the Pronunciation Key column and check whether you have said the word correctly.
3. Place a check (✓) mark in the column if you pronounced the word correctly.

Spelling Instructions

1. Have a peer dictate each medical term below using the Pronunciation Key column as a guide.
2. As each word is dictated, write it on a separate paper or enter it into a word-processing document.
3. Correct your spelling using the list below.
4. Place a check (✓) mark in the column if you pronounced the medical word correctly. Your instructor will then select 10 words for you to pronounce as a quiz.

Pronunciation Key	Medical Term	Pronounced Correctly ✓	Spelled Correctly ✓
ăm-nē-ō-sĕn-TĒ-sĭs	amniocentesis		
sē-SĀR-ē-ăn	cesarean		
kŏl-PŎS-kō-pē	colposcopy		
kū-rĕ-TĂZH	curettage		
dĭs-mĕn-ō-RĒ-ă	dysmenorrhea		
fŭl-gū-RĀ-shŭn	fulguration		
jĕs-TĀ-shŭn	gestation		
gī-nĕ-KŎL-ō-jĭst	gynecologist		
hē-mō-SĂL-pĭnks	hemosalpinx		
hĭs-tĕr-ĔK-tō-mē	hysterectomy		
ĭn-sŭ-FLĀ-shŭn	insufflation		
lăp-ăr-ŎS-kō-pē	laparoscopy		
mĕn-ĂR-kē	menarche		
mē-trō-TŌ-sĭs	metroptosis		
mŭl-TĬP-ă-ră	multipara		
ō-vā-rē-ō-RĔK-sĭs	ovariorrhexis		
ŏk-sē-TŌ-sĭn	oxytocin		
prī-mĭ-GRĂV-ĭ-dă	primigravida		
soo-dō-sī-Ē-sĭs	pseudocyesis		
pŭ-ĕr-PĒ-rē-ŭm	puerperium		

Your name: _____

Competency Verification

Number of correct pronunciations: _____ $\times$ 10
= _____ %
Number of correct spellings: _____ $\times$ 10
= _____ %

Pronunciation and Spelling Activity—Chapter 13: Endocrine System

Objective: To correctly spell and pronounce the medical terms in the table below

Pronunciation Instructions

1. Cover the Pronunciation Key column with a sheet of paper and say each word aloud.
2. Uncover the Pronunciation Key column and check whether you have said the word correctly.
3. Place a check (✓) mark in the column if you pronounced the word correctly.

Spelling instructions

1. Have a peer dictate each medical term below using the Pronunciation Key column as a guide.
2. As each word is dictated, write it on a separate paper or enter it into a word-processing document.
3. Correct your spelling using the list below.
4. Place a check (✓) mark in the column if you pronounced the medical word correctly. Your instructor will then select 10 words for you to pronounce as a quiz.

Pronunciation Key	Medical Term	Pronounced Correctly ✓	Spelled Correctly ✓
ăd-rēn-ō-MĔG-ă-lē	adrenomegaly		
KOR-tĭ-sōn	cortisone		
dī-ă-BĒ-tēz ĭn-SĬ-pĭ-dŭs	diabetes insipidus		
dī-ū-RĒ-sĭs	diuresis		
ē-LĔK-trō-līt	electrolyte		
ĕn-dō-krĭn-ŎL-ō-jē	endocrinology		
ĕk-sŏf-thăl-MŎM-ĕ-trē	exophthalmometry		
glī-kō-SŪ-rē-ă	glycosuria		
HŬR-sūt-ĭzm	hirsutism		
hō-mē-ō-STĀ-sĭs	homeostasis		
hī-drō-KOR-tĭ-sōn	hydrocortisone		
hī-pō-nă-TRĒ-mē-ă	hyponatremia		
ĭd-ē-ō-PĂTH-ĭk	idiopathic		
ĬN-sŭ-lĭn	insulin		
mī-krō-nū-rō-SĔR-jĕr-ē	microneurosurgery		
fē-ō-krō-mō-sī-TŌ-mă	pheochromocytoma		
pĭn-ē-ăl-ĔK-tō-mē	pinealectomy		
pŏl-ē-DĬP-sē-ă	polydipsia		
pŏl-ē-Ū-rē-ă	polyuria		
tŏks-ĭ-KŎL-ō-jĭst	toxicologist		

Your name: _____

Competency Verification

Number of correct pronunciations: _____ $\times$ 10
= _____ %
Number of correct spellings: _____ $\times$ 10
= _____ %

Pronunciation and Spelling Activity— Chapter 14: Nervous System

Objective: To correctly spell and pronounce the medical terms in the table below

Pronunciation Instructions

1. Cover the Pronunciation Key column with a sheet of paper and say each word aloud.
2. Uncover the Pronunciation Key column and check whether you have said the word correctly.
3. Place a check (✓) mark in the column if you pronounced the word correctly.

Spelling Instructions

1. Have a peer dictate each medical term below using the Pronunciation Key column as a guide.
2. As each word is dictated, write it on a separate paper or enter it into a word-processing document.
3. Correct your spelling using the list below.
4. Place a check (✓) mark in the column if you pronounced the medical word correctly. Your instructor will then select 10 words for you to pronounce as a quiz.

Pronunciation Key	Medical Term	Pronounced Correctly ✓	Spelled Correctly ✓
ă-sē-tă-MĬN-ō-fĕn	acetaminophen		
ăn-ăl-JĒ-zē-ă	analgesia		
ĂS-pĕr-ĭn	aspirin		
ăs-THĒ-nē-ă	asthenia		
brăd-ē-kĭ-NĒ-sē-ă	bradykinesia		
sĕ-RĒ-brăl PAWL-zē	cerebral palsy		
sĕr-ĕ-BRŎT-ō-mē	cerebrotomy		
dĭ-MĔN-shē-ă	dementia		
dĭs-LĔK-sē-ă	dyslexia		
lĕp-tō-mĕn-ĭn-GŎP-ă-thē	leptomeningopathy		
LĔTH-ăr-jē	lethargy		
măg-nĕt-ō-ĕn-cĕf-ă-LŎG-ră-fē	magnetoencephalography		
nū-RŎL-ĭs-ĭs	neurolysis		
nū-rō-TRĂNS-mĭt-ĕr	neurotransmitter		
păr-ĕs-THĒ-zē-ă	paresthesia		
pōl-ē-ō-mī-ĕl-Ī-tĭs	poliomyelitis		
sī-KĪ-ă-trē	psychiatry		
stĕr-ē-ō-TĂK-sĭk	stereotaxic radiosurgery		
sĭn-ĂL-jē-ă	synalgia		
SĬN-ăps	synapse		

Your name: _____

Competency Verification

Number of correct pronunciations: _____ $\times$ 10
= _____ %
Number of correct spellings: _____ $\times$ 10
= _____ %

Pronunciation and Spelling Activity—Chapter 15: Special Senses

Objective: To correctly spell and pronounce the medical terms in the table below

Pronunciation Instructions

1. Cover the Pronunciation Key column with a sheet of paper and say each word aloud.
2. Uncover the Pronunciation Key column and check whether you have said the word correctly.
3. Place a check (✓) mark in the column if you pronounced the word correctly.

Spelling Instructions

1. Have a peer dictate each medical term below using the Pronunciation Key column as a guide.
2. As each word is dictated, write it on a separate paper or enter it into a word-processing document.
3. Correct your spelling using the list below.
4. Place a (✓) mark in the column if you pronounced the medical word correctly. Your instructor will then pick 10 words for you to pronounce as a quiz.

Pronunciation Key	Medical Term	Pronounced Correctly ✓	Spelled Correctly ✓
ăm-blē-Ō-pē-ă	amblyopia		
blĕf-ă-rō-TŌ-sĭs	blepharoptosis		
kă-LĀ-zē-ŏn	chalazion		
kŏn-jŭnk-TĪ-văl	conjunctival		
ĕ-rĭth-rō-MĪ-sĭn	erythromycin		
ĕks-ŏf-THĂL-mŏs	exophthalmos		
gŏ-nē-ŌS-kŏ-pē	gonioscopy		
kĕr-ă-TŎT-ō-mē	keratotomy		
LĂB-ĭ-rĭnth	labyrinth		
LĂK-rĭ-mō-tōm	lacrimotome		
ŏk-ū-lō-mĭ-KŌ-sĭs	oculomycosis		
ŏl-FĂK-shŭn	olfaction		
ŏf-thăl-mō-dī-nă-MŎM-ĕ-trē	ophthalmodynamometry		
FĀK-ō-sēl	phacocele		
făk-ō-ē-MŪL-sĭ-fĭ-kā-shŭn	phacoemulsification		
fō-tō-PĬG-mĕnt	photopigment		
prĕz-bĭ-KŪ-sĭs	presbycusis		
tĭn-Ī-tŭs	tinnitus		
tĭm-pă-NŎS-tō-mē	tympanostomy		
vĭ-TRĔK-tō-mē	vitrectomy		

Your name: _____

Competency Verification

Number of correct pronunciations: _____ × 10
= _____ %
Number of correct spellings: _____ × 10
= _____ %

Supplemental Medical Record Activities

The following supplemental activities use common clinical scenarios to show how medical terminology is used to document patient care. Medical terms, their pronunciations, a medical record analysis, and an answer key are provided for the supplemental medical records activities. The following authentic medical reports are presented in a two-column style so your students have an opportunity to retype the report in an acceptable one-column format. All of the medical reports are correctly styled in the textbook and can be used as a reference to complete this activity. If you choose to have your students type and format the supplemental medical records in this Activity Pack, you can http://davisplus.fadavis.com/gylys/systems/.

■ ■ ■ Chapter 4–Body Structure

Supplemental Medical Record Activity 4–1

Radiology Report of the Skull, Facial Bones, and Orbits

Terminology

Terms in the table come from the medical record *Radiology Report of the Skull, Facial Bones, and Orbits* that follows. Use a medical dictionary such as *Taber's*

Cyclopedic Medical Dictionary, the appendices of Systems, 6th ed., or other resources to define each term. Then review pronunciations for each term and practice by reading the medical record aloud.

Term	Definition
anterior	
antrum ĂN-trŭm	
AP	
comminuted fracture KŎM-ĭ-nū-tĕd	
frontal sinus FRŬN-tăl SĬ-nŭs	
lateral LĂT-ĕr-ăl	
mandible MĂN-dĭ-bl	
oblique ō-BLĒK	
opaque ō-PĀK	
PA	
zygoma zĭ-GŌ-mă	

RADIOLOGY REPORT OF THE SKULL, FACIAL BONES, AND ORBITS

SKULL, FACIAL BONES, AND ORBITS: Standard skull series with lateral, PA, and Towne views as well as oblique and AP views of the mandible, base views of the zygoma. Waters view of the sinuses, and Reese views of the orbits were obtained. There is a comminuted fracture of the anterior wall of the frontal sinus with bone fragment protruding out into the soft tissues with marked swelling. In addition, the left zygoma is not seen on the base view except in the anterior and posterior portions, suggesting that it is fractured in its central portion with some depression. No other definite abnormality is seen. Repeat views of the zygoma and attempt to rotate the left zygoma out. The left maxillary sinus is slightly more opaque than the right, but no definite mass is seen and the bony walls appear intact. The walls of the orbit appear intact on the Reese views.

IMPRESSION:

1. Fracture of frontal sinus centrally with comminution.
2. Probable fracture of left zygoma.

3. Slight opacification of left maxillary antrum without definite fracture identified.

Analysis: Review the medical record *Radiology Report of the Skull, Facial Bones, and Orbits* to answer the following questions.

1. What four body structures were x-rayed?

   _____

2. What views were included in the skull series?

   _____

3. What is a comminuted fracture?

   _____

4. How did the physician come to the conclusion that the zygoma was fractured in its central portion?

   _____

Supplemental Medical Record Activity 4–2

Gunshot Wound to the Chest

Terminology

Terms in the table come from the medical record *Gunshot Wound to the Chest* that follows. Use a medical dictionary such as *Taber's Cyclopedic Medical*

Dictionary, the appendices of *Systems,* 6th ed., or other resources to define each term. Then review pronunciations for each term and practice by reading the medical record aloud.

Term	Definition
cannulate KĂN-ū-lāt	
comatose KŌ-mă-tōs	
contused kŏn-TOOZD	
diaphoretic dī-ă-fō-RĔT-ĭk	
diaphragm DĪ-ă-frăm	
inferior vena cava VĒ-nă KĀ-vă	
intercostal space ĭn-tĕr-KŎS-tăl	
pericardial sac pĕr-ĭ-KĂR-dē-ăl	

Term	Definition
pericardial tamponade pĕr-ĭ-KĂR-dē-ăl tăm-pŏn-ĀD	
posterolateral pŏs-tĕr-ō-LĂT-ĕr-ăl	
right quadrant KWŎD-rănt	
sternum STĔR-nŭm	
superior vena cava VĒ-nă KĀ-vă	
ventricle VĔN-trĭ-kl	

GUNSHOT WOUND TO THE CHEST

This 18-year-old-white female presented to the emergency department with a gunshot wound to her left chest. The bullet entered at approximately the fifth intercostal space just to the left of the sternum. From the bevel of the bullet trajectory and the powder burn, it can be seen to enter the right-to-left trajectory on an axis pointing from the anterior right chest to the posterior left flank. This trajectory carried the bullet in a direct path through the heart. The bullet appears to be lodged in the left posterior back.

Upon admission, the patient was not comatose but obviously quite pale and diaphoretic, with what appeared to be a pericardial tamponade. Her blood pressure was low; her pulse rate was rapid. It did not appear that she had any other wounds.

Emergency precautions were taken to include insertion of a left chest tube and three IV lines: one superior vena caval line, one inferior vena caval line, and a left arm line. The right groin was used to cannulate the femoral vessel with an Intracath under direct vision. All this was accomplished quite rapidly. She was stable. A chest film was obtained to note the trajectory of the bullet; it appeared it might be in the area of the spleen. Therefore, a right quadrant tap was done. No blood was obtained and no fluid was obtained, and she was taken to the operating room at that time, since the operating crew was then prepared.

The operative note will follow in separate dictation, but briefly what was found was a bullet wound entering in approximately the fifth intercostal space, passing what appeared to be through the pericardial sac, creasing the left ventricle in two spaces. It was the anterior portion of the left ventricle on the lateral portion of the heart that was injured. The bullet passed through this area and lodged in the left flank in a posterolateral position. The diaphragm was not violated. It was, therefore, not opened and the abdomen was then not explored. The lingula of the lung was also lacerated as the bullet passed by it. It was bleeding actively, as was the heart. There was a pericardial tamponade. This was relieved when the pericardium was widely opened, the heart being delivered and suturing undertaken. The active bleeding in the heart was stopped by placing a finger over the hole and suturing the heart closed over Teflon pledgets. There was a great deal of macerated muscle on the anterior surface of the heart, and therefore it was quite difficult to place the pledgets accurately. This was done, one on each side of the bullet hole; large doubled pledgets were used because single pledgets could not support the muscle adequately. There appeared to be an area of about 3.5 cm of nonviable or very contused heart muscle. All this having been accomplished, her blood pressure was stabilized and she was brought to the intensive care unit. Nothing else is known about this patient at this time. Her family will be spoken to.

Analysis: Review the medical record *Gunshot Wound to the Chest* to answer the following questions.

1. Where did the bullet enter the patient's body?

   _____

2. What direction did the bullet travel through the body?

   _____

3. Where does the bullet appear to be lodged?

_____

4. Was the diaphragm injured?

_____

5. How did the physician stop the active bleeding of the heart?

_____

■ ■ ■ Chapter 5–Integumentary System

Supplemental Medical Record Activity 5–1

Pigmented Solar Keratosis

Terminology

Terms in the table come from the medical record *Pigmented Solar Keratosis* that follows. Use a medical dictionary such as *Taber's Cyclopedic Medical*

Dictionary, the appendices of *Systems*, 6th ed., or other resources to define each term. Then review pronunciations for each term and practice by reading the medical record aloud.

Term	Definition
cherry angioma ăn-jē-Ō-mă	
excoriated acne ĕks-KŌ-rē-ā-tĭd ĂK-nē	
idiopathic guttate hypomelanosis ĭd-ē-ō-PĂTH-ĭk GOO-tāt hĭ-pō-mĕl-ă-NŌ-sĭs	
photo-protection fō-tō-prō-TĔK-shŭn	
pigmented solar keratosis PĬG-mĕnt-ĕd SŌ-lăr kĕr-ă-TŌ-sĭs	
seborrheic keratosis sĕb-ō-RĒ-ĭk kĕr-ă-TŌ-sĭs	

PIGMENTED SOLAR KERATOSIS

Dear Doctor Rosen:

Ms. Bassett presents for a "skin cancer check." She readily volunteers that she has spent a considerable amount of time out in the sun, although there is no family history of skin cancer.

I reassured the patient about typical changes of so-called "idiopathic guttate hypomelanosis" over her legs, plus a solitary seborrheic keratosis on her left wrist and a single cherry angioma over her left thigh.

Checking the sun-exposed sites, I did detect an early pigmented solar keratosis over her right zygoma. She also has numerous excoriated acne lesions on her face. I elected to freeze this precancer with liquid nitrogen on an applicator after stressing the importance of photoprotection.

Ms. Bassett will return as required.

Analysis: Review the medical record *Pigmented Solar Keratosis* to answer the following questions.

1. What was the predisposing factor causing the patient's present condition?

   _____

2. What did the doctor recommend to the patient to prevent future problems with solar keratosis?

   _____

3. What treatment was performed on the precancerous lesions?

   _____

4. When does the doctor want to see the patient again?

   _____

Supplemental Medical Record Activity 5–2

Severe Pressure Ulcer, Left Foot, Now Gangrenous

Terminology

Terms in the table come from the medical record *Severe Pressure Ulcer, Left Foot, Now Gangrenous* that follows. Use a medical dictionary such as *Taber's Cyclopedic*

Medical Dictionary, the appendices of *Systems*, 6th ed., or other resources to define each term. Then review pronunciations for each term and practice by reading the medical record aloud.

Term	Definition
AK	
amputation ăm-pū-TĀ-shŭn	
arteriosclerosis ăr-tē-rē-ō-sklĕ-RŌ-sĭs	
contractures kŏn-TRĂK-chŭrz	
debridement dā-brēd-MŎN	
flexion FLĔK-shŭn	
gangrenous GĂNG-grĕn-ŭs	
Pressure ulcer	

SEVERE PRESSURE ULCER, LEFT FOOT, NOW GANGRENOUS

PAST HISTORY: This 84-year-old white male, a patient at Geriatric Hospital, with multiple problems, including generalized arteriosclerosis, has had increasing problems with left heel pressure ulcer over several months. Initially, local care and debridement seemed to be improving this problem along with physical therapy and good padding. However, due to the patient's severe senile mental state and acquired flexion contractures of the lower extremities, it has been increasingly difficult to keep pressure off of the heel, and finally the heel and the remainder of the foot began to break down and are now gangrenous. Consultation with Dr. Larry Fisher was obtained at my request, and his recommendation was above-knee amputation. This was discussed with the patient's daughter, who is his conservator, and she agrees.

EXAMINATION OF THE EXTREMITIES: There is rigidity of all extremities, but in the lower extremities there are essentially flexion contractures. The left foot is quite dark with a large pressure ulcer on the heel and generalized infection of the foot. Pulses are not palpable. There is a smaller pressure ulcer on the right heel but the remainder of the foot is in good shape.

PLAN: Admit patient to surgery for AK amputation.

Analysis: Review the medical record *Severe Pressure Ulcer, Left Foot, Now Gangrenous* to answer the following questions.

1. What measures did the health-care providers initially use to lessen the problems caused by heel pressure?

_____

2. Why was it difficult for the patient to keep pressure off the heel?

_____

3. What type of contractures did the physician identify?

_____

4. Was the right foot as bad as the left?

_____

5. What type of amputation did the doctor perform?

_____

■ ■ ■ Chapter 6–Digestive System

Supplemental Medical Record Activity 6–1

Esophagogastroduodenoscopy with Biopsy

Terminology

Terms in the table come from the medical record *Esophagogastroduodenoscopy with Biopsy* that follows. Use a medical dictionary such as *Taber's Cyclopedic*

Medical Dictionary, the appendices of *Systems,* 6th ed., or other resources to define each term. Then review pronunciations for each term and practice by reading the medical record aloud.

Term	Definition
antral ĂN-trăl	
EGD	
endoscopy ĕn-DŎS-kō-pē	
epigastric ĕp-ĭ-GĂS-trĭk	
erythematous ĕr-ĭ-THĔM-ă-tŭs	
esophagitis ē-sŏf-ă-JĪ-tĭs	
esophagoscope ē-SŎF-ă-gō-skōp	
fundus FŬN-dŭs	
Helicobacter hĕl-ĭ-kō-BĂK-tĕr	
IV	
mg	

Term	Definition
oropharynx or-ō-FĂR-ĭnks	
retroflex RĔ-trō-flĕks	
squamocolumnar junction skwā-mō-kō-LŬM-năr JŬNK-shŭn	
ulceration ŭl-sĕr-Ā-shŭn	

ESOPHAGOGASTRODUODENOSCOPY WITH BIOPSY

PREOPERATIVE DIAGNOSIS: Chronic epigastric pain of unknown origin.

POSTOPERATIVE DIAGNOSIS:
1. Mild antral gastritis.
2. Distal esophagitis.

PROCEDURE: Esophagogastroduodenoscopy with biopsy.

ANESTHESIA: Cetacaine spray. Demerol 50 mg; Versed 4 mg IV.

INDICATIONS: Chronic epigastric pain.

SUMMARY OF PROCEDURE: This 55-year-old white male was informed of the nature of the procedure, its associated risks, possible benefits, and alternatives. He was given an opportunity to ask questions prior to the procedure. The Pentax video upper endoscope was gently placed in the oropharynx and guided under direct vision into the proximal esophagus. The endoscope was advanced easily to the third portion of the duodenum. The duodenal mucosa was unremarkable in appearance. The endoscope was gradually withdrawn to the duodenal bulb, revealing no abnormalities. The endoscope was withdrawn through the pylorus. The antrum was examined. The antrum was diffusely erythematous with a salt-and-pepper–type appearance and breakup of light reflex consistent with mild gastritis. A biopsy was taken for a *Helicobacter* test. The body of the stomach was unremarkable. Retroflex view of the cardia and fundus revealed no abnormalities. The endoscope was straightened and withdrawn to the gastroesophageal junction. The squamocolumnar junction was irregular in contour. There was a single long mucosal break consistent with grade A esophagitis. No actual ulceration was seen. As

the endoscope was gradually withdrawn, a tubular view of the body of the esophagus revealed normal mucosa.

Patient tolerated the procedure well and there were no complications. He was observed until stable and then discharged to the care of his companion with instructions not to eat or drink for an hour and not to drive or perform tasks requiring concentration for the remainder of the day.

RECOMMENDATIONS:
1. Await result of biopsy for *Helicobacter*.
2. Continue Propulsid.
3. Prevacid 30 mg by mouth daily.

Analysis: **Review the medical record *Eophagogastroduodenoscopy with Biopsy* to answer the following questions.**

1. What anesthetic was administered for this procedure?

   _____

2. What type of endoscope was used for the procedure?

   _____

3. How far was the endoscope placed in the GI tract?

   _____

4. Why was a biopsy performed?

   _____

5. Were ulcers found in the mucosa?

   _____

6. What was the final diagnosis?

   _____

Supplemental Medical Record Activity 6–2

Fissure-in-Ano

Terminology

Terms in the table come from the medical record *Fissure-in-Ano* that follows. Use a medical dictionary such as *Taber's Cyclopedic Medical Dictionary*, the appendices of *Systems*, 6th ed., or other resources to define each term.

Term	Definition
defecation dĕf-ĕ-KĀ-shŭn	
epidural anesthesia ĕp-ĭ-DOO-răl ăn-ĕs-THĒ-zē-ă	
excision ĕk-SĬ-zhŭn	
external hemorrhoids HĔM-ō-roydz	
fissure-in-ano FĬS-ūr ĭn-Ā-nō	
fissurectomy fĭsh-ūr-ĔK-tō-mē	
hemogram HĒ-mō-grăm	
internal hemorrhoids HĔM-ō-roydz	
microscopic mī-krō-SKŎ-pĭc	
morbid obesity MOR-bĭd ō-BĒ-sĭ-tē	
sentinel pile SĔN-tĭn-ĕl PĪ-ĕl	
urinalysis ū-rĭ-NĂL-ĭ-sĭs	

FISSURE-IN-ANO

ADMITTING DIAGNOSIS: Fissure-in-ano.

DISCHARGE DIAGNOSIS: Fissure-in-ano, improved. External and internal hemorrhoids, improved.

OPERATION: Fissurectomy with excision of sentinel hemorrhoid.

DISPOSITION: Home and office care.

DISCHARGE MEDICATION: Darvocet-N, 100, one every 4 hours as required for pain.

This 29-year-old man had severe pain on defecation for 2 months. Examination revealed a chronic posterior fissure. This had failed to respond to conservative measures, and he entered the hospital for fissurectomy.

Physical examination was unremarkable except for morbid obesity of 350 pounds. Hemogram and urinalysis were within normal limits, with the exception of a few bacteria on microscopic examination of his urine and a trace of hemoglobin in the urine.

On the day of admission, under epidural anesthesia, the rectum and anus were explored, and he was found to have a chronic fissure with a sentinel pile as well as mixed internal and external hemorrhoids. The sentinel pile and fissure were excised and the anal canal dilated. Patient's postoperative course was uneventful. He is improved and dismissed to home and office care.

Analysis: Review the medical record *Fissure-in-Ano* to answer the following questions.

1. How long had this patient been having pain?

_____

2. What word in this report is synonymous with pile?

_____

3. In what part of the anus was the fissure located?

_____

4. How is morbid obesity defined?

_____

5. What did the doctor do to the patient's anal area following excision of the fissure?

_____

Supplemental Medical Record Activity 6–3

Inguinal Hernia

Terminology

Terms in the table come from the medical record *Inguinal Hernia* that follows. Use a medical dictionary such as *Taber's Cyclopedic Medical Dictionary,* the appendices of *Systems,* 6th ed., or other resources to define each term. Then review pronunciations for each term and practice by reading the medical record aloud.

Term	Definition
bilaterally bī-LĂT-ĕr-ăl-lē	
hernia HĔR-nē-ă	
hesitancy HĔS-ĭ-tĕn-sē	
inguinal ĬNG-gwĭ-năl	
laparoscopic lăp-ă-rō-SKŎP-ĭc	
micturition mĭk-tū-RĬ-shŭn	
prostatitis prŏs-tă-TĪ-tĭs	
testes TĔS-tēs	
umbilicus ŭm-BĬL-ĭ-kŭs	
varicocele VĂR-ĭ-kō-sēl	

INGUINAL HERNIA

Dear Doctor McFee:

Thank you for allowing us to see Arthur Anthony on November 22, 20xx. He is a 51-year-old newspaper mailer who had an incidental finding of a left inguinal hernia on physical exam. Since then he has had increased fullness and an occasional heavy sensation in the left groin. About 15 years ago he underwent left varicocele repair, and no hernia was noted at that time. He admits to no known precipitating event. Occasionally he has difficulty initiating micturition, having urinary hesitancy and occasional frequency. He has recently completed treatment of prostatitis from you and these symptoms have resolved. Mr. Anthony has also had long-standing swelling just above the umbilicus.

On examination, a definite hernia is present in the left inguinal canal adjacent to the pubic tubercle. This easily reduces. There is no corresponding abnormality in the right groin. Testes are bilaterally descended, no masses or tenderness are present. His left varicocele incision has healed nicely with a nearly unperceivable scar. Umbilical hernia is present which cannot be completely reduced.

I agree that Mr. Anthony has a left inguinal hernia. We talked about the advantages and risks of conventional versus laparoscopic repair. It is reasonable to undergo laparoscopic repair. He is at increased risk for injury to his testicular blood supply because of his previous varicocele repair and will be scheduled for the laparoscopic repair. I will keep you informed as additional information becomes available.

Analysis: Review the medical record *Inguinal Hernia* to answer the following questions.

1. How did the patient discover he had a hernia?

   _____

2. What two symptoms did the patient experience?

   _____

3. How was the urination of the patient described?

   _____

4. Which two treatments were described to repair the hernia?

   _____

5. Which method of repair did the physician recommend?

   _____

■ ■ ■ Chapter 7–Respiratory System

Supplemental Medical Record Activity 7–1

Asthma (Child)

Terminology

Terms in the table come from the medical record *Asthma (Child)* that follows. Use a medical dictionary such as *Taber's Cyclopedic Medical Dictionary*, the appendices of *Systems*, 6th ed., or other resources to define each term. Then review pronunciations for each term and practice by reading the medical record aloud.

Term	Definition
aerosolized ĔR-ō-sō-līzd	
albuterol ăl-BŪ-tĕr-ăl	
asthma ĂZ-mă	
expiratory wheeze ĕks-PĪ-ră-tor-ē HWĒZ	

Term	Definition
organomegaly or-gă-nō-MĔG-ă-lē	
ventilated VĔN-tĭ-lā-tĕd	

Asthma (Child)

HISTORY: According to his parents, this is one of several Pope Memorial Hospital admissions for this 27-month-old male with asthma since birth. He has had multiple hospitalizations for asthma. He has previously not been ventilated. He was well until yesterday when he developed cough and increased work of breathing. He was treated with aerosolized albuterol at home. He was taken to Travis Medical Facility today, where he was quite tight. He initially received two albuterol aerosols and then went to x-ray. He came back again quite tight and received a total of five albuterol aerosols with some improvement. He received 30 mg of prednisone orally in the emergency department. He was then transferred without difficulty. There is a family history on the mother's side for asthma. There is no other significant family history.

The patient's previous medical history is unremarkable other than his asthma. His usual medicines are Intal and albuterol with Pulmo-Aide. The remainder of the past medical history, family history, and review of systems is unremarkable.

PHYSICAL EXAMINATION: Well-developed, well-nourished male in moderate respiratory distress.

HEENT: Tympanic membranes unremarkable. Eyes, nose, mouth, and throat normal.

NECK: Without masses. Supple.

LUNGS: Breath sounds clear bilaterally with somewhat decreased air exchange and diffuse expiratory wheeze. Work of breathing is mildly to moderately increased.

ABDOMEN: Soft and nontender without organomegaly or mass.

GU: Normal male.

EXTREMITIES: Unremarkable.

NEUROLOGICAL: He is alert and appropriate. Cranial nerves intact. Reflexes 2+ and symmetrical.

ASSESSMENT: Two-year-old male with asthma, moderately severe.

PLAN: I will treat him with IV Solu-Medrol and IV cefuroxime and aerosolized albuterol and Tornalate. Consider continuous albuterol if he does not improve with intermittent aerosol.

Analysis: Review the medical record *Asthma (Child)* to answer the following questions.

1. How long has this child had a history of asthma?

   _____

2. Why was the child returned to Pope Memorial Hospital after being treated earlier at Travis Medical Facility?

   _____

3. What medication did the child receive in the emergency department?

   _____

4. What contributory factors might be significant for this child's illness?

   _____

5. What type of lung sounds were heard upon examination?

   _____

Supplemental Medical Record Activity 7–2

Bronchoscopy

Terminology

Terms in the table come from the medical record *Bronchoscopy* that follows. Use a medical dictionary such as *Taber's Cyclopedic Medical Dictionary*, the appen-dices of *Systems*, 6th ed., or other resources to define each term. Then review pronunciations for each term and practice by reading the medical record aloud.

Term	Definition
biopsies BĪ-ŏp-sēz	
bronchoscope BRŎNG-kō-skōp	
bronchoscopy brŏng-KŎS-kō-pē	
brushings BRŬSH-ĭngz	
carina kă-RĪ-nă	
endotracheal lesion ĕn-dō-TRĀ-kē-ăl LĒ-zhŭn	
epiglottis ĕp-ĭ-GLŎT-ĭs	
infiltration ĭn-fĭl-TRĀ-shŭn	
mass	
medially MĒ-dē-ăl-lē	
mg	
mL	
nasotracheal tube nă-zō-TRĀ-kē-ăl	
occluded ō-KLŪ-dĭd	
saturation săt-ū-RĀ-shŭn	

BRONCHOSCOPY

PREOPERATIVE DIAGNOSIS: Left lung mass.

POSTOPERATIVE DIAGNOSIS: Left lung mass.

OPERATION: Bronchoscopy.

ANESTHESIA: Infiltration of 10 mL of 0.1% Xylocaine.

PREOPERATIVE MEDICATIONS: Demerol 75 mg and 0.6 mg of atropine. The patient also received a total of 4 mg of Versed intravenously just prior and during the operation.

PROCEDURE: The bronchoscopy was performed. A nasotracheal tube was inserted into the right nostril while the patient was receiving the supplemental oxygen through the left nostril, and the saturation, which was being monitored closely, did not fall below 94% at any time.

FINDINGS: The epiglottis was normal. The vocal cords were normal, with normal closure on phonation. The trachea was normal without endotracheal lesion or external tracheal compression, and the carina was sharp and clear.

Right Lung: The right mainstem bronchus, the bronchus of the right upper lobe, right lower lobe, and right middle lobe, with all segments and subsegments identified. There were some moderate whitish secretions in the right lower lobe bronchus which were suctioned clear. There was no endobronchial lesion or external bronchial compression seen in the right lung.

Left Lung: The mid to lower section of the left mainstem bronchus was displaced anteriorly and medially; this was also partly occluded by a combination of an external bronchial tumor which was eroded into the left mainstem bronchus. There was a 50% obstruction of the left mainstem bronchus, but the bronchoscope could be passed beyond the obstruction and the left lower lobe bronchus, with all segments and subsegments identified.

Multiple biopsies, washings, and brushings were obtained from the left mainstem bronchus tumor.

There was some bleeding around the tumor, even before the bronchoscope was advanced to the tumor, which was washed.

ESTIMATED BLOOD LOSS: Approximately 5 cubic centimeters.

Analysis: Review the medical record *Bronchoscopy* to answer the following questions.

1. Refer to Figure 7-1 to locate the trachea and bronchi. How far was the bronchoscope inserted?

   _____

2. What was the color of the secretions in the right lower lobe of the lung?

   _____

3. What was the finding regarding the right lung?

   _____

4. In which part of the left lung was the mass identified?

   _____

5. What was obtained from the left mainstem bronchus tumor?

   _____

Supplemental Medical Record Activity 7–3

Peritonsillar Abscess

Terminology

Terms in the table come from the medical record *Peritonsillar Abscess* that follows. Use a medical dictionary such as *Taber's Cyclopedic Medical*

Dictionary, the appendices of *Systems,* 6th ed., or other resources to define each term. Then review pronunciations for each term and practice by reading the medical record aloud.

Term	Definition
cervical adenopathy SĔR-vĭ-kăl ăd-ĕ-NŎP-ă-thē	
edema ĕ-DĒ-mă	
erythema ĕr-ĭ-THĒ-mă	
erythematous ĕr-ĭ-THĔM-ă-tŭs	

Term	Definition
mucopurulent mū-kō-PŪR-ū-lĕnt	
nasopharyngitis nā-zō-făr-ĭn-JĪ-tĭs	
oropharynx or-ō-FĂR-ĭnks	
peritonsillar abscess pĕr-ĭ-TŎN-sĭ-lăr ĂB-sĕs	
pharyngitis făr-ĭn-JĪ-tĭs	
purulent PŪR-ū-lĕnt	
rhinoscopy rī-NŎS-kō-pē	
submandibular sŭb-măn-DĬB-ū-lăr	
tonsillectomy tŏn-sĭl-ĔK-tō-mē	

PERITONSILLAR ABSCESS

Dear Doctor Masters:

RE: Sandra Gomez

I had the opportunity of seeing your patient today, a student at the University of Toledo College of Health Science and Human Service, who has a history of recurrent pharyngitis and peritonsillar abscess. She developed a sore throat and fever over this past weekend, was seen Monday at Health Services, and was placed on Pen-Vee K Although her fever has diminished, she is having increasing throat pain and cervical adenopathy reminiscent of her episode of peritonsillar abscess. She presents for ENT consultation.

She currently is on penicillin and Ortho-Novum. She is not known to be allergic to any medications and states herself to otherwise be in good health.

Her examination shows obvious swelling of the left submandibular lymph node. There is no overlying skin erythema. The oropharynx shows enlargement of the left tonsil; however, there is no evidence of edema of the palate or pharyngeal wall. Jaw range of motion is normal. The nasopharyngeal examination shows mucopurulent nasal drainage with erythematous inflammation of the adenoid pad. Anterior rhinoscopy shows no evidence of purulent nasal drainage.

IMPRESSION:
1. Nasopharyngitis
2. History of peritonsillar abscess.
3. No current evidence to suggest peritonsillar abscess.

RECOMMENDATIONS:
1. Switch to Augmentin from penicillin.
2. Ibuprofen as needed for pain.
3. Return as needed.
4. Agree with plan for tonsillectomy in December.

Analysis: Review the medical record *Peritonsillar Abscess* to answer the following questions.

1. What type of recurrent illness was identified in the patient's medical history?

   _____

2. Where was the noticeable swelling?

   _____

3. What did the nasopharyngeal examination show?

   _____

4. Was the drainage the same inside the nose?

   _____

5. What was the immediate treatment?

   _____

Supplemental Medical Record Activity 7–4

Allergic rhinitis

Terminology

Terms in the table come from the medical record *Allergic Rhinitis* that follows. Use a medical dictionary such as *Taber's Cyclopedic Medical Dictionary*, the appendices of *Systems*, 6th ed., or other resources to define each term. Then review pronunciations for each term and practice by reading the medical record aloud.

Term	Definition
exacerbates ĕks-ĂS-ĕr-bātz	
hypertrophy hī-PĔR-trŏ-fē	
nasopharynx nā-zō-FĂR-ĭnks	
otoscopic ō-tō-SKŎP-ĭc	
rhinitis rī-NĪ-tĭs	
rhinorrhea rī-nō-RĒ-ă	
septoplasty SĔP-tō-plăs-tē	
turbinate TŬR-bĭn-āt	

ALLERGIC RHINITIS

Dear Doctor Gardner:

I had the pleasure of seeing Ms. Lopez today for complaints suggestive of allergic rhinitis. She has had a long history of nasal obstruction. Previously she was found to have mechanical destruction secondary to septal deformity and turbinate hypertrophy. She had a septoplasty and turbinate reduction the latter part of last year, which has significantly improved her airway compromise. She has noted some seasonal nasal symptoms (sneezing, watery rhinorrhea) as well as a tickling of the palate and burning of the eyes. This typically exacerbates in the spring and summer months. She is just beginning to experience the symptoms again at this time. She has nothing that would suggest recurrent sinusitis.

Her examination today revealed unremarkable otoscopic findings. Nasal exam reveals an essentially midline septum with improvement in the nasal airway following septoplasty. The turbinates remain lateralized inferiorly. The mucosa, however, throughout the nasal cavities appears to be somewhat pale and edematous with a serous discharge present. The sinuses are nontender. The nasopharynx was clear. The oral cavity and oropharynx were without mucosal lesion or induration. Neck is unremarkable to palpation. My impression, based on her symptoms and findings, is allergic rhinitis. I have given samples of Double Strength Vancenase AQ and Allegra for this; however, I think it would be best to see an allergist to undergo definitive allergy testing.

Analysis: Review the medical record *Allergic Rhinitis* to answer the following questions.

1. What surgeries did the patient have last year?

_____

2. What was the outcome of last year's surgery?

_____

3. What seasonal symptoms are currently noted by the patient?

_____

4. How is the nasal mucosa described?

_____

5. What was the recommendation of the physician?

_____

■ ■ ■ Chapter 8–Cardiovascular System

Supplemental Medical Record Activity 8–1

Cardiomyopathy and Supraventricular Arrhythmias

Terminology

Terms in the table come from the medical record _Cardiomyopathy and Supraventricular Arrhythmias_ that follows. Use a medical dictionary such as _Taber's_ _Cyclopedic Medical Dictionary,_ the appendices of _Systems,_ 6th ed., or other resources to define each term. Then review pronunciations for each term and practice by reading the medical record aloud.

Term	Definition
angiography ăn-jē-ŎG-ră-fē	
arrhythmias ă-RĬTH-mē-ăz	
atherosclerosis ăth-ĕr-ō-sklĕ-RŌ-sĭs	
bradyarrhythmias brăd-ē-ă-RĬTH-mē-ăz	
bundle branch block	
cardiomegaly kăr-dē-ō-MĔG-ă-lē	
claudication klaw-dĭ-KĀ-shŭn	
diaphoresis dī-ă-fō-RĒ-sĭs	
differential dĭf-ĕr-ĔN-shăl	
echocardiography ĕk-ō-kăr-dē-ŎG-ră-fē	
embolus ĔM-bō-lŭs	
fibrillation fĭ-brĭl-Ā-shŭn	
hypercholesterolemia hī-pĕr-kō-lĕs-tĕr-ŏl-Ē-mē-ă	

Term	Definition
hypertension hī-pĕr-TĔN-shŭn	
icterus ĬK-tĕr-ŭs	
palpitations păl-pĭ-TĀ-shŭnz	
petechiae pē-TĔ-kē-ē	
PMI	
PT	
PTT	
syncope SĬN-kō-pē	
transient ischemic attack TRĂN-sē-ĕnt ĭs-KĒ-mĭk ă-TĂK	

CARDIOMYOPATHY AND SUPRAVENTRICULAR DYSRHYTHMIAS

HISTORY

CHIEF COMPLAINT: Episode of nausea, diaphoresis, palpitations, and near syncope.

PRESENT ILLNESS: Mr. Mayfield is a 49-year-old man with a complicated medical cardiac history. He underwent an angiography in 20xx and was told that he should be treated with medical therapy. He was seen at Presbyterian General Hospital in the past for atrial fibrillation and treated with digoxin. He was first seen at El Camino Hospital in March 20xx when he had an episode of rapid atrial fibrillation associated with probably systemic embolus to his abdomen. At that point in time, he underwent an echocardiography showing a dilated aortic root and subsequent CT scan of the chest confirmed an aortic root of 6 cm with the ascending root being 4.5 cm. Subsequently, catheterization showed he had normal coronary arteries, dilated left ventricle and sinuses, and an enlarged aortic root with only mild aortic insufficiency.

The patient was seen by multiple surgical consultants here at Presbyterian, at El Camino Hospital, and at Stanford. He ultimately underwent composite replacement of his aortic valve and aortic root by Dr. Robert Terhune at El Camino Hospital due to his dilated ascending aortic root and the fear he would at some point in time develop acute aortic dissection or death if this aortic root continued to expand.

He has been followed for his cardiomyopathy and supraventricular arrhythmias and ventricular arrhythmias on medical therapy, and he has really done quite well until recently when he has had several distinct episodes of the sudden onset of nausea, diaphoresis, and palpitations with his feeling that he is "going to go out," although he has not had any frank syncope. He had an episode today like the one that occurred at K-Mart and came to the emergency department. He is being admitted to the hospital for observation and further workup for potential causes of his presyncopal episodes.

In terms of his risk factors for potential underlying cardiovascular disease, he has a family history of atherosclerosis but no history of smoking, hypertension, diabetes, or hypercholesterolemia. He has never had a history of rheumatic fever, heart murmur, transient ischemic attack, cerebrovascular accident, or claudication.

PAST HISTORY: History of testicular carcinoma treated with orchiectomy and radiation therapy.

ALLERGIES: None.

MEDICATIONS: See Present Illness.

HABITS: No history of smoking or excess alcohol intake.

FAMILY HISTORY: Atherosclerosis.

REVIEW OF SYSTEMS

PHYSICAL EXAMINATION

GENERAL: A lert, pleasant male in no acute distress.

VITAL SIGNS: Heart rate 88, blood pressure 154/108.

INTEGUMENT: No petechiae or rash.

HEENT: No icterus.

CHEST: Clear lung fields with no wheezes, rhonchi, rales, or rubs.

CARDIAC: There are 5 cubic centimeters of jugular venous distention. Carotids are 2+ and equal bilaterally without bruits. PMI is in the sixth inter-costal space in the midclavicular line. There are crisp valve sounds and a grade 1/6 murmur at the apex but no S3, opening snap, ejection click, or diastolic murmur.

ABDOMEN: Soft, with normal bowel sounds. There is no mass, rebound, or tenderness. Liver is 8 cm in the midclavicular line. I cannot feel the spleen.

GU: Deferred.

EXTREMITIES: Trace right and left ankle edema. No calf tenderness.

CNS: Grossly within normal limits.

LABORATORY DATA:
1. Complete blood count, differential, sodium, BUN, creatinine, potassium, PT, and PTT are pending.
2. Chest x-ray shows cardiomegaly and upper lobe redistribution consistent with volume overload.
3. EKG shows sinus rhythm with left bundle branch block and left atrial enlargement.

IMPRESSION:
1. Presyncope.
2. History of paroxysmal atrial fibrillation and ventricular dysrhythmias in the past.
3. Cardiomyopathy.
4. Status post aortic semilunar valve replacement and aortic arch repair for dilated aortic root.
5. History of testicular carcinoma, treated with orchiectomy and radiation therapy.

PLAN: This 49-year-old man has a history of cardiomyopathy, paroxysmal atrial fibrillation, and ventricular dysrhythmias in addition to replacement of his aortic valve and repair of his aortic arch for dilated aortic root. He has had several distinct episodes of nausea, diaphoresis, palpitations, and pre-syncope without frank loss of consciousness, and he is being admitted to the hospital tonight for observation for any potential ventricular or bradydysrhythmias as possible etiology of his symptoms.

He will be seen in consultation by Dr. Munier of the electrophysiology service for consideration of elec-trophysiological testing, possible tilt table testing, to rule out vasovagal episodes and/or significant ven-tricular arrrhythmias as an etiology of his symptoms.

Analysis: **Review the medical record *Cardiomyopathy and Supraventricular Arrhythmias* to answer the following questions.**

1. Why was Mr. Mayfield treated with digoxin following his evaluation at Presbyterian Hospital?

   _____

2. What was the probable cause of the episode of rapid atrial fibrillation when Mr. Mayfield was first seen at El Camino Hospital?

   _____

3. Refer to Figure 8-2. Notice the location of the aorta and the aortic semilunar valve. What procedure did Dr. Robert Terhune perform?

   _____

4. Why was the patient admitted following his examination in the emergency department?

   _____

5. What family history, if any, may have contributed to the patient's problems?

   _____

6 What tests will Dr. Munier perform?

   _____

Supplemental Medical Record Activity 8–2

Coronary Artery Disease with Myocardial Infarction

Terminology

Terms in the table come from the medical record *Coronary Artery Disease with Myocardial Infarction* that follows. Use a medical dictionary such as *Taber's* *Cyclopedic Medical Dictionary*, the appendices of *Systems*, 6th ed., or other resources to define each term. Then review pronunciations for each term and practice by reading the medical record aloud.

Term	Definition
bypass graft surgery BĪ-păs GRĂFT SŪR-jĕr-ē	
coronary angiography KOR-ō-nă-rē ăn-jē-ŎG-ră-fē	
CPK	
ischemic cardiomyopathy ĭs-KĒ-mĭc kăr-dē-ō-mī-ŎP-ă-thē	
laparotomy lăp-ăr-ŎT-ō-mē	
myocardial infarction mī-ō-KĂR-dē-ăl ĭn-FĂRK-shŭn	
occlusion ō-CLOO-shŭn	
stenosis stĕ-NŌ-sĭs	
ventricular and supraventricular arrhythmias vĕn-TRĬK-ū-lăr, soo-pră-vĕn-TRĬK-ū-lăr ă-RĬTH-mē-ăz	

CORONARY ARTERY DISEASE WITH MYOCARDIAL INFARCTION

HISTORY

PRESENT ILLNESS: This 77-year-old man was hospitalized at Crescent City Hospital with chest pain, where a diagnosis of myocardial infarction was made. The patient had CPK elevation to 800 units per liter. The patient was subsequently discharged home and, within 24 hours, he was rehospitalized because of heart failure and cardiac arrhythmia. The patient was transferred to University of California Hospital in San Francisco for further cardiac evaluation. He underwent cardiac catheterization and coronary angiography. His ejection fraction was around 30% to 35%. He has severe left main coronary artery stenosis and right coronary artery occlusion.

The patient had a laparotomy in October 20xx for bowel obstruction. The patient had a carcinoid tumor resected 4 or 5 years ago. During recent laparotomy, he was found to have diffuse carcinoid involvement of the liver and mesentery. The patient did have small-bowel resection. He now has a colostomy. The patient is expected to live 2 to 3 years.

PAST HISTORY: History of long-standing hypertension. The patient has colostomy for diverticular bleeding in 20xx. He has had transurethral resection of the prostate. He had recent small bowel resection for bowel obstruction from carcinoid tumor. He has had previous transient ischemic attack. He has bilateral carotid disease with 60% to 70% stenoses.

PHYSICAL EXAMINATION

GENERAL: Exam reveals an alert, oriented male who has had recent weight loss.

VITAL SIGNS: Blood pressure 120/70, pulse 80 per minute, respirations and temperature normal.

HEAD AND NECK: Normal except for faint bilateral carotid bruits. No lymphadenopathy.

CHEST: Clear.

HEART: Regular rhythm. No murmur.

ABDOMEN: Soft. No mass or tenderness. Bowel sounds present.

EXTREMITIES: He has palpable femoral and posterior tibial pulses bilaterally.

IMPRESSION:

1. Severe coronary artery disease with recent myocardial infarction, high-grade left main coronary artery stenosis and occlusion of right coronary artery, ischemic cardiomyopathy, ventricular and supraventricular dysrhythmias.
2. History of carcinomatosis, status post recent bowel obstruction, previous colostomy for diverticular bleeding.
3. Carotid occlusive disease with history of previous transient ischemic attack.

RECOMMENDATION: The patient and his family are fully aware of cardiac catheterization findings. Dr. Kastanis has also discussed the situation with the patient. The patient is in agreement with proceeding with coronary artery bypass graft surgery, knowing that he has abdominal carcinomatosis. However, the patient is expected to live for 2 to 3 years from carcinoid tumor. His overall operative risk is around 10%. In view of his multiple medical problems, I will not aggressively pursue carotid angiogram prior to his coronary artery bypass graft surgery. Informed consent has been obtained for the operation.

Analysis: Review the medical record *Coronary Artery Disease with Myocardial Infarction* to answer the following questions.

1. What diagnosis was made at Crescent City Hospital?

   _____

2. Why was the patient readmitted?

   _____

3. What information did the cardiac catheterization provide?

   _____

4. To what extent are the carotids blocked?

   _____

5. What is his anticipated life expectancy based on his history of cancer?

   _____

6. What procedure will be performed?

   _____

■ ■ ■ Chapter 9–Blood, Lymph, and Immune Systems

Supplemental Medical Record Activity 9–1

Bone marrow study following chemotherapy

Terminology

Terms in the table come from the medical record *Bone Marrow Study Following Chemotherapy* that follows. Use a medical dictionary such as *Taber's Cyclopedic Medical Dictionary,* the appendices of *Systems,* 6th ed., or other resources to define each term. Then review pronunciations for each term and practice by reading the medical record aloud.

Term	Definition
basophilic bā-sō-FĬL-ĭk	
CBC	
G-CSF	

Term	Definition
intraoperative radiotherapy ĭn-tră-ŎP-ĕr-ă-tĭv rā-dē-ō-THĔR-ă-pē	
leukocytosis loo-kō-sī-TŌ-sĭs	
myelosuppression mĭ-ĕ-lō-sŭ-PRĔSH-ŭn	
neuroblastoma nū-rō-blăs-TŌ-mă	
occult ŏ-KŬLT	
orthochromatophilic or-thō-krō-măt-ō-FĬL-ĭk	
polychromatophilic pŏl-ē-krō-măt-ō-FĬL-ĭk	
segs	

BONE MARROW STUDY FOLLOWING CHEMOTHERAPY

CLINICAL NOTE: Patient is a 2-year-old boy with an abdominal neuroblastoma that has been undergoing very aggressive therapy since September 20xx. The patient has had several laparotomies and one course of intraoperative radiotherapy and is currently being strongly considered for bone marrow transplant again at University of California San Francisco. Bone marrow aspirate is being done to rule out the appearance of any occult neuroblastoma in his bone marrow.

LABORATORY: CBC done on the day before the procedure, 10/25/xx, revealed a white count of 28,900, hemoglobin 8.4, hematocrit 27.8, platelets 45,000 with a differential of 80% segs, 2.2% lymphocytes, 15% monocytes. It should be noted that the patient had just finished a course of G-CSF and this accounts for the leukocytosis.

WRIGHT STAIN BONE MARROW: Wright stains of the bone marrow aspirate obtained from both the right and left posterior iliac crest revealed a very cellular specimen that is very active and indicative of a recovery marrow. All cell lines are present and there is normal differentiation of all cell lines, but there is an increased percentage of monocytes and promyelocytes seen in the marrow. Extensive review of the marrow from both the right and left side, looking at several slides, fails to reveal any obvious neuroblastoma rosettes or tumor clumps.

A 200-cell differential is as follows: blasts 2%, lymphocytes 8%, monocytes 16.5%, megakaryocytes 0.5%, preerythroblasts 6.5%, basophilic normoblasts 6.5%, polychromatophilic normoblasts 18%, orthochromatophilic normoblasts 1.5%, promyelocytes 9%, myelocytes 14%, metamyelocytes 6%, bands 7.5%, segmented neutrophils 4.5%.

DIAGNOSTIC IMPRESSION: This is an M1 active marrow, demonstrating recovery from recent myelosuppression and the effect of G-CSF with no evidence of malignancy.

ADDENDUM: It should be noted that 8 cc of heparinized marrow was sent to Dr. Seeger's Lab at Children's Hospital in Los Angeles for monoclonal antibody assessment to seek any occult neuroblastoma.

Analysis: Review the medical record *Bone Marrow Study Following Chemotherapy* to answer the following questions.

1. What procedures were previously performed on the patient?

   _____

2. Why was a bone marrow aspirate performed on the patient?

   _____

3. What appears to have caused the patient's leukocytosis?

   _____

4. What was the result of the Wright stain bone marrow study?

5. Why was a sample of heparinized bone marrow sent to Dr. Seeger's laboratory?

Supplemental Medical Record Activity 9–2

Stage III-A Hodgkin Disease

Terminology

Terms in the table come from the medical record *Stage III-A Hodgkin Disease* that follows. Use a medical dictionary such as *Taber's Cyclopedic Medical Dictionary,* the appendices of *Systems,* 6th ed., or other resources to define each term. Then review pronunciations for each term and practice by reading the medical record aloud.

Term	Definition
Hodgkin disease HŎJ-kĭn dĭ-ZĒZ	
megakaryocytes mĕg-ă-kăr-ē-ō-sītz	
monos MŎN-ōs	
morphological examination mor-fō-LŎJ-ĭk-ăl	
neutropenia noo-trō-PĒ-nē-ă	
segs sĕgz	
spicules SPĬK-ūlz	
thrombocytopenia thrŏm-bō-sī-tō-PĒ-nē-ă	

STAGE III-A HODGKIN DISEASE

CLINICAL HISTORY: Patient has a stage III-A Hodgkin disease, finishing her chemotherapy many weeks ago. She has persistent neutropenia and thrombocytopenia since her chemotherapy. Marrow examination is done to rule out bone marrow involvement with her Hodgkin disease.

PERIPHERAL BLOOD: Peripheral blood sample furnished on 10/13/xx showed a white count of 11,200, hemoglobin 11.2, hematocrit 35.8, platelets 160,000 (increase from 44,000 2 days before), with 89% segs, 2.6% bands, 7.8% monos; morphological examination was not performed.

BONE MARROW: Marrow technique is adequate. Stain is adequate. Significant spicules are seen for evaluation. Representatives of all nuclear cell lines are seen in adequate numbers for evaluation. Megakaryocytes appear normal to increased in numbers. There is myeloid predominance. Of a 200-cell differential, 26% of the cells represent erythroid precursors, 2% represent lymphoid precursors, with the remainder representing all elements of the myeloid series. There appears to be an increased percentage of myelocytes and metamyelocytes in numerous areas of the smear. No malignant cells of extramedullary elements are noted.

IMPRESSION: Normal bone marrow aspirate without evidence of malignant disease. Myeloid predominance.

Analysis: Review the medical record *Stage III-A Hodgkin Disease* to answer the following questions.

1. Why was a bone marrow examination performed on this patient?

_____

2. What was noted in the peripheral blood regarding platelets?

_____

3. In the bone marrow aspirate, what was the predominant cell observed?

_____

4. What was the impression regarding malignancy?

_____

■ ■ ■ **Chapter 10–Musculoskeletal System**

Supplemental Medical Record Activity 10–1

Spinal stenosis

Terminology

Terms in the table come from the medical record *Spinal Stenosis* that follows. Use a medical dictionary such as *Taber's Cyclopedic Medical Dictionary,* the appendices of *Systems,* 6th ed., or other resources to define each term. Then review pronunciations for each term and practice by reading the medical record aloud.

Term	Definition
concentric annular disk bulge kŏn-SĔN-trĭk ĂN-ū-lăr DĬSK	
conus medullaris KŌ-nŭs mĕd-ū-LĂR-ĭs	
facet arthropathy FĂS-ĕt ăr-THRŎP-ă-thē	
intervertebral disk degeneration ĭn-tĕr-VĔRT-ĕ-brĕl DĬSK dē-gĕn-ĕr-Ā-shŭn	
L2	
MRI	
osteophyte ŎS-tē-ō-fīt	
paraspinous pără-SPĪ-nŭs	
spinal stenosis SPĪ-năl stĕ-NŌ-sĭs	
T1	
thecal sac THĒ-kăl SĂK	

SPINAL STENOSIS

MRI STUDY: Lumbar spine.

CLINICAL INFORMATION: Low back pain. Right leg pain.

TECHNIQUE: 2 MRI series (sagittal T2, axial T1).

FINDINGS: No abnormal retroperitoneal or paraspinous soft-tissue masses are seen. The size and position of the conus medullaris appear normal.

L2-3: There is concentric annular disk bulge and accompanying marginal osteophyte. There is mild ventral flattening of the thecal sac. There is mild to moderate degree of acquired spinal stenosis. Facet arthropathy contributes to this.
L3-4: There is concentric annular disk bulge. There is mild ventral flattening of the thecal sac.
L4-5: There is intervertebral disk degeneration and concentric annular disk bulge. There is mild ventral flattening of the thecal sac.
L5-S1: There is intervertebral disk degeneration.

IMPRESSION: Mild to moderate central canal spinal stenosis at L2-3.

Analysis: Review the medical record *Spinal Stenosis* to answer the following questions.

1. Why was this patient referred to x-ray?

_____

2. What kind of thecal sac flattening was evident in the L2-3 vertebral view?

_____

3. At what levels was intervertebral disk degeneration noted?

_____

4. What did the MRI reveal at L5-S1?

_____

5. Where is the conus medullaris located?

_____

Supplemental Medical Record Activity 10–2

Neck and Shoulder Pain Due to Auto Accident

Terminology

Terms in the table come from the medical record *Neck and Shoulder Pain Due to Auto Accident* that follows. Use a medical dictionary such as *Taber's Cyclopedic*

Medical Dictionary, the appendices of *Systems,* 6th ed., or other resources to define each term. Then review pronunciations for each term and practice by reading the medical record aloud.

Term	Definition
C4	
craniotomy krā-nē-ŎT-ō-mē	
degenerative disk disease dē-GĔN-ĕr-ă-tĭv DĬSK	
exacerbation ĕks-ăs-ĕr-BĀ-shŭn	
L5	
modalities mō-DĂL-ĭ-tēz	
physical therapy FĬZ-ĭ-kăl THĔR-ă-pē	
S1	

Neck and Shoulder Pain Due to Auto Accident

Patient is a 58-year-old female whom I saw for orthopedic evaluation subsequent to a motor vehicle accident which occurred September 29, 20xx. She was initially seen by me 2 years earlier, on July 17, 20xx, at which time she was complaining of neck and left shoulder area pain. She had a long history of neck area symptomatology subsequent to the development of cancer for which she has undergone radical neck dissection with pectoralis transfer, as well as a craniotomy procedure in the past. She subsequently has undergone surgery for excision of bone fragment and abscess formation and had eye surgery, all as a consequence of the cancer. At the time of my initial examination, x-rays showed degenerative disk disease at the C4-5 and C5-6 levels. I had recommended conservative treatment and modalities and felt that she would have gradual improvement subsequent to her motor vehicle accident. She was also having some lower back discomfort. X-rays had shown some degenerative disk disease at the L5-S1 level. I saw her for reevaluation on September 6, and at that time she was improving, indicating left neck stiffness and improvement with respect to the lower back discomfort. I had discharged her from clinic at that time, although I recommended that she return on an as-needed basis. She was seen again 9 months later on June 6, 20xx, for the neck, left shoulder area, and lower back. At that time, she was complaining of right hip and right heel pain. She had indicated a subsequent injury whereby a bus on which she was riding ran into a pole, causing her to develop lower back symptomatology. I recommended a short course of physical therapy and had instructed her to return to clinic in 2 weeks' time for reassessment. The patient failed to return for her subsequent visits. Her present symptomatology is unknown to me. At the time of her last visit, I had recommended that a possible treatment alternative could include cortisone injection into the area of maximal tenderness over the right iliac crest. Treatment was deferred pending completion of her physical therapy program. There are no records available from the physical therapist, and I therefore do not know whether she in fact had the physical therapy as was recommended for her. Should the patient return for reevaluation, we would be better able to delineate her present symptomatology.

In response to your letter of February 14, 20xx, at the time of her September 29, 20xx, motor vehicle accident, she was complaining of neck, left shoulder, and lower back symptomatology. Her prognosis was good in that she underwent conservative treatment and modalities and had initial improvement. At the time of her most recent evaluation, she was complaining of pain primarily in the lower back.

Her present back symptomatology would be a combination of the most recent accident as well as exacerbation of the prior motor vehicle accident and also exacerbation subsequent to her extensive neck injury.

Conservative treatment and modalities were recommended to her. She would not have been considered a surgical candidate based upon the motor vehicle accident as described.

Patient had marginal strength and motion subsequent to her neck cancer and subsequent surgery. The motor vehicle accident would have exacerbated this prior condition necessitating the subsequent treatment.

Analysis: **Review the medical record** *Neck and Shoulder Pain Due to Auto Accident* **to answer the following questions.**

1. Was the motor vehicle accident the primary cause of the patient's neck pain?

   _____

2. What types of surgery did the patient have as a result of the cancer?

   _____

3. Why is it difficult for the physician to evaluate the patient's present condition?

   _____

4. What was the status of the patient's neck mobility prior to the motor vehicle accident?

   _____

Supplemental Medical Record Activity 10–3

Chronic Tendinitis

Terminology

Terms in the table come from the medical record *Chronic Tendinitis* that follows. Use a medical dictionary such as *Taber's Cyclopedic Medical Dictionary*, the appendices

of *Systems*, 6th ed., or other resources to define each term. Then review pronunciations for each term and practice by reading the medical record aloud.

Term	Definition
capitellum kăp-ĭ-TĚL-ŭm	
chondromalacia kŏn-drō-măl-Ā-shē-ă	
condylar KŎN-dĭ-lăr	
dissection dĭ-SĔK-shŭn	
exsanguinating ĕks-SĂNG-gwĭn-ā-tĭng	
hemostasis hē-mō-STĀ-sĭs	
oblique ō-BLĒK	
phlebitis flĕ-BĪ-tĭs	
prophylactic prō-fĭ-LĂK-tĭk	
purulent PŪR-ū-lĕnt	
recalcitrant rē-CĂL-sĭ-trănt	
supracondylar soo-pră-KŎN-dĭ-lăr	
tendinitis tĕn-dĭn-Ī-tĭs	
tourniquet TOOR-nĭ-kĕt	

CHRONIC TENDINITIS

PREOPERATIVE DIAGNOSIS: Chronic tendinitis, right elbow.

POSTOPERATIVE DIAGNOSIS: Chronic tendinitis, right elbow.

OPERATION: Nirschl procedure, right elbow.

SURGEON: Van Acker, M.D.

INDICATIONS: Patient is a 59-year-old man with recalcitrant tendinitis of his right elbow. This involved both the medial and lateral condylar surfaces. Conservative care consisted of corticosteroid injections, physical therapy, exercises, and anti-inflammatories. He has had an elbow sleeve. It was suggested that he undergo the above procedure in the hopes of decreasing elbow pain. The risks of the procedure, including infection, phlebitis, neurovascular and tendon injuries, anesthetic complications, failure of the procedure, recurrence, inadequate result, and anesthetic problems, among others, were discussed and accepted.

PROCEDURE: Patient was brought to the operating room and given a general anesthetic. He was given prophylactic Kefzol 1-gram push. The tourniquet was placed on the proximal aspect of the right arm. The arm was scrubbed, prepped, and draped in a routine sterile fashion. After exsanguinating the limb, the tourniquet was elevated to 250 mm Hg.

An oblique skin incision was made beginning along the lateral supracondylar ridge and extending to the radial head. Hemostasis was obtained with the Bovie on the lateral condyle. This was carefully incised, the ECRB tendon was exposed, and findings showed typical chronic tendinitis. It was sent to histology for pathological analysis.

Dissection was deep to include a lateral arthrotomy. The radial head of the articular surface of the capitellum was visualized and intact. There was some straw-colored, not purulent, synovial fluid in the joint. There were no loose bodies. The joint was irrigated, checking for chondromalacia pathology and there was none. Satisfied with the procedure, the wound was closed. Patient was returned to the recovery room. Recovery was unremarkable.

ESTIMATED BLOOD LOSS: Approximately 5 cubic centimeters.

Analysis: Review the medical record *Chronic Tendinitis* to answer the following questions.

1. How was the tendinitis described?

   _____

2. What conservative treatment had the patient undergone prior to surgery?

   _____

3. What complications were described to the patient?

   _____

4. After the arm was scrubbed and draped, what procedure was undertaken?

   _____

5. What was the finding after incision?

   _____

6. How was the synovial fluid described?

   _____

■ ■ ■ Chapter 11–Genitourinary System

Supplemental Medical Record Activity 11–1

Testicular Mass

Terminology

Terms in the table come from the medical record *Testicular Mass* that follows. Use a medical dictionary such as *Taber's Cyclopedic Medical Dictionary,* the appendices of *Systems,* 6th ed., or other resources to define each term. Then review pronunciations for each term and practice by reading the medical record aloud.

Term	Definition
alpha-fetoprotein ĂL-fă FĒ-tō-prō-tēn	
anorexia ăn-ō-RĔK-sē-ă	
epididymis ĕp-ĭ-DĬD-ĭ-mĭs	

Term	Definition
fluctuance FLŬK-chū-ănts	
GU	
HCG	
hydrocele HĪ-drō-sēl	
inhomogeneous ĭn-hō-mō-JĒ-nē-ŭs	
malaise mă-LĀZ	
mg	
phallus FĂL-ŭs	
urethral ū-RĒ-thrăl	
voiding VOY-dĭng	

TESTICULAR MASS

HISTORY

REASON FOR ADMISSION: Right testicular mass.

HISTORY OF PRESENT ILLNESS: Patient is a healthy 23-year-old man who, 2 months ago, noted a right testicular pain radiating to his right groin and right flank. After approximately 1 month of these symptoms, he was seen at the Student Health Service at University of California Santa Cruz, where he is a student, and was diagnosed as having an infection in the epididymis and was treated with doxycycline. He had subsequent improvement in both pain and swelling over the course of the first few days; however, the pain then returned with mild increase in swelling again. He also reports a few episodes of chills for the past month; however, he denies anorexia, malaise, night sweats, trauma, any abnormal voiding symptoms, or urethral discharge. He is sexually active.

PAST MEDICAL HISTORY: Unremarkable.

SURGERY: None.

MEDICATIONS:
1. Penetrex 400 mg by mouth twice a day.
2. Ibuprofen 800 mg as required for pain.

SOCIAL HISTORY: He drinks alcohol moderately and is a nonsmoker.

FAMILY HISTORY: Negative.

PHYSICAL EXAMINATION

GU: Penis, normal phallus without lesions. Testes descended bilaterally. The left testicle is entirely normal in consistency and size. The right testicle is approximately two times the size of the left. It is hard, without any areas of fluctuance. It is only mildly tender. The epididymis does not feel enlarged. There was no hydrocele. There is no groin adenopathy.

A scrotal ultrasound was done in Santa Cruz the day before yesterday, which revealed an inhomogeneous right testicular mass consistent with tumor versus possible abscess.

IMPRESSIONS: Rule out right testicular tumor versus possible abscess.

PLAN: Admit the patient this evening for right inguinal exploration with possible radical orchiectomy. We also plan to proceed with chest x-ray, preoperative lab work including alpha-fetoprotein and beta HCG.

INFORMED CONSENT: The patient is scheduled for the above surgery on 1/23/xx. The indications, risks, and alternatives of the procedure were explained in detail to both him and his parents. The risks include bleeding, infection, and testicular loss. He understands the above and has no further questions and agrees to proceed with surgery.

Analysis: Review the medical record *Testicular Mass* to answer the following questions.

1. What were the patient's initial symptoms?

   _____

2. What was the patient initially treated for?

   _____

3. Did the patient have a urethral discharge?

   _____

4. What did the scrotal ultrasound reveal?

   _____

5. What type of surgery is planned for the patient?

   _____

Supplemental Medical Record Activity 11–2

Monilial-Type Balanitis

Terminology

Terms in the table come from the medical record *Monilial-Type Balanitis* that follows. Use a medical dictionary such as *Taber's Cyclopedic Medical Dictionary,* the appendices of *Systems,* 6th ed., or other resources to define each term. Then review pronunciations for each term and practice by reading the medical record aloud.

Term	Definition
Accu-Chek ĂK-ū-chĕk	
chlamydia klă-MĬD-ē-ă	
cultures KŬL-chŭrz	
dysuria dīs-Ū-rē-ă	
foreskin FOR-skĭn	
frequency FRĒ-qwĕn-cē	
GC	
herpes HĔR-pēz	
hypoglycemic agents hī-pō-glī-SĒ-mĭk Ā-jĕnts	
monilial-type balanitis mō-NĬL-ē-ăl bă-lă-NĪ-tĭs	
uncircumcised ŭn-SĔR-kŭm-sīzd	
urgency ĔR-jĕn-sē	

MONILIAL-TYPE BALANITIS

HISTORY

CHIEF COMPLAINT: Peeling skin on penis.

HISTORY OF PRESENT ILLNESS: Patient is a 50-year-old male who presents to the emergency department with chief complaint of peeling skin on his penis for the last 3 weeks. The patient has attempted to remedy this with Vaseline and baby oil. It has not improved. The patient denies any dysuria, frequency, or urgency. He denies any abdominal pain. He denies any rectal pain.

PAST MEDICAL HISTORY: Glucose intolerance. The patient states that he has been on oral hypoglycemic agents in the past. He has since run out. He does not have a primary care physician.

PHYSICAL EXAMINATION

GENERAL APPEARANCE: This is a well-developed, well-nourished male in minimal acute distress.

VITAL SIGNS: Normal.

GU: Both testicles are descended. The patient has no hernias. The patient is uncircumcised. The patient's foreskin is retracted. The patient appears to have monilial-type balanitis.

The patient has an Accu-Chek of 312. Since the patient does not have a primary care physician, urinalysis was sent. Cultures were sent for GC, chlamydia, and herpes.

PLAN: See discharge instructions.

Analysis: Review the medical record *Monilial-Type Balanitis* to answer the following questions.

1. What prompted the patient to seek medical care?

   _____

2. Did the patient have any urinary problems?

   _____

3. Was the patient taking medications for his glucose intolerance?

   _____

4. Why did the doctor order cultures?

   _____

■ ■ ■ Chapter 12–Female Reproductive System

Supplemental Medical Record Activity 12–1

Intrauterine Pregnancy

Terminology

Terms in the table come from the medical record *Intrauterine Pregnancy* that follows. Use a medical dictionary such as *Taber's Cyclopedic Medical Dictionary,* the appendices of *Systems,* 6th ed., or other resources to define each term. Then review pronunciations for each term and practice by reading the medical record aloud.

Term	Definition
ab	
amnionitis ăm-nē-ō-ō-NĪ-tĭs	
cesarean section sē-SĀR-ē-ăn SĔK-shŭn	
effaced ĕ-FĀST	
footling breech FOOT-lĭng BRĒCH	

Term	Definition
gestation jĕs-TĀ-shŭn	
gravida GRĂV-ĭ-dă	
para PĂR-ă	
spontaneous abortion spŏn-TĀ-nē-ŭs ă-BOR-shŭn	

INTRAUTERINE PREGNANCY

HISTORY OF PRESENT ILLNESS: Patient is a 27-year-old gravida 3, para 1, Ab 1 female with last menstrual period April 7, 20xx, and estimated date of confinement of January 11, 20xx, who is currently at 31 to 32 weeks' gestation with an uncomplicated pregnancy until 12:30 p.m., November 9, when she experienced spontaneous premature rupture of membranes. She was started on terbutaline pump. However, on the morning of November 10 at approximately 4:30 a.m. she had onset of regular uterine contractions. She presented to Methodist Hospital and had a temperature of 100.2°F degrees. She was started on magnesium sulfate, ampicillin, and gentamicin and was transferred to Mt. Sinai Hospital. Examination prior to transfer revealed the cervix to be 3 cm dilated and completely effaced with footling breech presentation. Complete blood count prior to transfer revealed hemoglobin 11.2, hematocrit 32.8, platelets 209,000, and white count 12,000.

Past obstetrical history includes spontaneous abortion ×1 and vaginal delivery of a 6-pound, 3-ounce infant following uncomplicated pregnancy.

PAST MEDICAL HISTORY: Negative.

PHYSICAL EXAMINATION:

GENERAL: The patient is alert, well oriented, in no acute distress. Vital signs are within normal limits, except her temperature is 100°F degrees.

ABDOMEN: Gravid with bilateral lower quadrant tenderness over the uterus to palpation. The liver is not palpable. Fetal heart tones are in the 150s and are reactive per external monitor.

PELVIC: Not repeated.

PRENATAL LABS: On August 10, blood type O positive, rubella immune, hepatitis B surface antigen negative. AFP normal on September 14. Pap smear on August 12 class one.

IMPRESSION:
1. Intrauterine pregnancy at 31+ weeks.
2. Premature rupture of membranes.
3. Preterm labor.
4. Amnionitis.
5. Breech presentation.

PLAN: We did proceed with delivery by primary cesarean section. The possible need for vertical uterine incision and the implications for future pregnancies were discussed with the patient and her husband.

Analysis: **Review the medical record *Intrauterine Pregnancy* to answer the following questions.**

1. What happened to this patient on November 9?

   _____

2. Was the patient term when labor started?

   _____

3. What was the indication for cesarean section?

   _____

4. How many times was the patient pregnant?

   _____

Supplemental Medical Record Activity 12–2

Labor Examination in Adolescent Mother

Terminology

Terms in the table come from the medical record *Labor Examination in Adolescent Mother* that follows. Use a medical dictionary such as *Taber's Cyclopedic Medical* *Dictionary*, the appendices of *Systems*, 6th ed., or other resources to define each term. Then review pronunciations for each term and practice by reading the medical record aloud.

Term	Definition
anemic ă-NĒ-mĭk	
effaced ĕ-FĀST	
gestation jĕs-TĀ-shŭn	
ischial spines ĬS-kē-ăl	
primigravida prī-mĭ-GRĂV-ĭ-dă	
promontory PRŎM-ŏn-tōr-ē	
vertex VĔR-tĕks	

LABOR EXAMINATION IN ADOLESCENT MOTHER

PHYSICAL EXAMINATION

GENERAL: Patient is a 16-year-old single primigravida with a due date of January 20. She spontaneously broke her bag of water at 9 a.m., began having contractions at 10 a.m., and was admitted at 12:15, 3 to 4 cm with 3- to 4-minute contractions. The patient was fairly comfortable with this. Prenatal record has been reviewed. This is the patient's first trip to the hospital. She denies any serious heart and lung disorder or any previous significant medical history.

Laboratory studies are remarkable only in that she has been anemic, with initial hematocrit of 30% with the pregnancy. Hemoglobin was repeated at 32 weeks' gestation after the patient had been on oral iron three times daily, and I do not see the results of the second repeat on the chart.

VITAL SIGNS: BP: 110/70. Pulse: 100°F. Temperature: 36.6.

BREASTS: Full and soft without obvious masses.

ABDOMEN: Soft. Estimated fetal weight 7 pounds.

PELVIC: Exam at 1:30 p.m. reveals the cervix to be 6 to 7 cm, vertex at −2, cervix completely effaced and the pelvis is contracted. The ischial spines are quite sharp, directed inward toward the midportion of the pelvis. Sacrum is flattened. I can touch the promontory at 11 to 11.5 cm.

I would say that there is a definite risk of this not passing the midplane of the pelvis.

Analysis: Review the medical record *Labor Examination in Adolescent Mother* to answer the following questions.

1. Why was the patient admitted to the hospital?

   _____

2. What is the patient doing for her anemia?

   _____

3. Does the doctor feel the patient will be able to have a vaginal delivery?

   _____

■ ■ ■ **Chapter 13–Endocrine System**

Supplemental Medical Record Activity 13–1

Primary Hyperparathyroidism

Terminology

Terms in the table come from the medical record *Primary Hyperparathyroidism* that follows. Use a medical dictionary such as *Taber's Cyclopedic Medical Dictionary*, the appendices of *Systems*, 6th ed., or other resources to define each term. Then review pronunciations for each term and practice by reading the medical record aloud.

Term	Definition
alkaline phosphatase ĂL-kǎ-lĭn FŎS-fǎ-tāz	
bilateral urolithiasis bī-LĂT-ĕr-ǎl ū-rō-lǐ-THĪ-ǎ-sǐs	
hyperlipidemia hī-pĕr-lǐp-ǐ-DĒ-mē-ǎ	
hyperparathyroidism hī-pĕr-pǎr-ǎ-THĪ-roy-dǐzm	
phosphorus FŎS-fō-rǔs	
serum calcium SĒ-rǔm KĂL-sē-ǔm	

PRIMARY HYPERPARATHYROIDISM

This 65-year-old patient presented today for follow-up evaluation of his primary hyperparathyroidism. As you know, the patient's serum calcium has remained in a good range. The most recent calcium I have is 10.7 from February 14, 20xx. Phosphorus was low at 2.2, and alkaline phosphatase was high at 181, presumably reflecting the hyperparathyroid state.

The patient tells me he has now been diagnosed as having bilateral urolithiasis, more marked on the left than the right. As you know, the patient had a 24-hour urine for calcium when I initially saw him in mid 20xx, and the value was 158 mg per 24 hours despite calcium supplementation.

On examination, blood pressure is 124/62, pulse is 88, and weight is 146 pounds (10-pound weight loss over the past year). No cervical changes noted. Lungs are clear. Cardiac examination is unremarkable. Extremities are benign.

Medications consist only of Lopid twice a day.

IMPRESSION:
1. Primary hyperparathyroidism.
2. Recent episode of urolithiasis.
3. Hyperlipidemia.
4. Abnormal alkaline phosphatase.

The urolithiasis is very disturbing. I have asked the patient to repeat his 24-hour urine calcium and to obtain a 24-hour urine for uric acid as well. The patient will be calling to discuss these results. A bone scan may be appropriate in view of the rising alkaline phosphatase. Although the patient's bone density from 1 year ago was in the nonosteoporotic range, if there are other signs that the patient's hyperparathyroidism is producing significant adverse skeletal effects or has precipitated the episode of urolithiasis, then a parathyroidectomy would be an appropriate recommendation.

Analysis: Review the medical record *Primary Hyperparathyroidism* to answer the following questions.

1. Refer to Figure 13-1. Where are the parathyroid glands located?

_____

2. What important function does parathyroid hormone (PTH) perform?

_____

3. In which way is the increase of PTH affecting this patient?

_____

4. What are the target organs of PTH? (Refer to Table 13-3.)

_____

■ ■ ■ Chapter 14–Nervous System

Supplemental Medical Record Activity 14–1

Peripheral Neuropathy

Terminology

Terms in the table come from the medical record _Peripheral Neuropathy_ that follows. Use a medical dictionary such as _Taber's Cyclopedic Medical_ _Dictionary,_ the appendices of _Systems,_ 6th ed., or other resources to define each term. Then review pronunciations for each term and practice by reading the medical record aloud.

Term	Definition
arthralgias ăr-THRĂL-jē-ŭz	
EMG	
encephalitis ĕn-sĕf-ă-LĪ-tĭs	
gait gāt	
meningitis mĕn-ĭn-JĪ-tĭs	
otosclerosis ō-tō-sklĕ-RŌ-sĭs	
peripheral neuropathy pĕr-ĬF-ĕr-ăl nū-RŎP-ă-thē	
proprioception prō-prē-ō-SĔP-shŭn	

Peripheral Neuropathy

CLINICAL HISTORY: This 61-year-old divorced white female who is on disability has a history of prolonged pain and burning in her feet, more on the left than the right initially, now equally; diminished proprioception; and the sense of difficulty in walking, particularly in the dark. This all began 2½ to 3 years ago.

She has additionally been diagnosed apparently as having lupus erythematosus, seen by a military physician who suggested the diagnosis and referred her to Dr. Reed, who apparently confirmed in 20xx. She recalls that she had an elevated sedimentation rate at 45 years of age but does not recall other elements of lab abnormality.

She has some moderate intermittent low back pain, and has less of the burning in the lower extremities but still some numbness which is increased by sitting, driving, or walking for too long a time.

She has no history of head or neck injury, meningitis, or encephalitis. The only family history of neurological illness is that her maternal grandmother had some type of seizure disorder.

NEUROLOGICAL EXAMINATION:

HEAD AND NECK: Normal configuration, full range of head and neck movements and no audible bruits.

CRANIAL NERVE EXAMINATION: Reveals symmetrical function of cranial nerves II through XII except for hearing loss.

MOTOR SYSTEM EXAMINATION: Reveals normal gait and station and generally good strength, coordination, and reflexes. Forward flexion brings her fingertips down to her toes, but when she tries to straighten up, she then bends her legs at the knees, says that she could not get up otherwise.

SENSORY EXAMINATION: Reveals decreased position and vibratory sense as well as pinprick in the lower extremities, much more on the right up to the upper third of the shin, and just in the foot and ankle on the left.

IMPRESSION: Peripheral neuropathy of unknown cause. Possibly related to lupus but it does not strike me that she has other major clinical manifestations at this time. There is nothing that suggests central nervous system lupus at this juncture either. Additionally, she has low back pain, intermittent diffuse arthralgias easily controlled by minimal medication, and otosclerosis with hearing loss.

PLANS: She should have EMG and nerve conduction studies of the lower extremities to further characterize the nature and progression of her neuropathy, and will arrange this with my associate.

Analysis: **Review the medical record** *Peripheral Neuropathy* **to answer the following questions.**

1. What are the patient's presenting complaints?

   _____

2. Are the patient's cranial nerves intact?

   _____

3. How was the motor system examination described?

   _____

4. How extensive is the patient's sensory loss?

   _____

Supplemental Medical Record Activity 14–2

Facial Paralysis

Terminology

Terms in the table come from the medical record *Facial Paralysis* that follows. Use a medical dictionary such as

Taber's Cyclopedic Medical Dictionary, the appendices of *Systems,* 6th ed., or other resources to define each term. Then review pronunciations for each term and practice by reading the medical record aloud.

Term	Definition
brainstem BRĀN-stĕm	
cerebellar sĕr-ĕ-BĚL-ăr	
dysarthric dĭs-ĂR-thrĭc	
EEG	
facial paralysis FĀ-shăl pă-RĂL-ĭ-sĭs	
MRI	

Term	Definition
nystagmus nĭs-TĂG-mŭs	
uvula Ū-vū-lă	

FACIAL PARALYSIS

NEUROLOGICAL EXAMINATION

GENERAL APPEARANCE: This is an elderly female lying in bed, alert and awake, and fairly cooperative. Speech was fluent and not dysarthric. Comprehension was fairly preserved. She was oriented to place and person but disoriented to time. Her memory for recent and past events was severely impaired. She could not provide any information concerning her past medical history.

CRANIAL NERVES: Full visual fields to confrontation. Optic disks are sharp. Extraocular movements are full in all directions; there was no nystagmus. Both pupils were reactive to light. Facial sensation was intact. There was a left facial weakness which seemed to be of peripheral type, but this could not be determined with certainty. The uvula was in the midline. Gag reflex was intact. Tongue was in the midline.

CEREBELLAR FUNCTION: Cerebellar function could not be tested due to her inability to follow two-step commands.

MOTOR: Normal muscle tone and normal strength throughout. There was no focal limb weakness.

SENSORY: Intact pinprick and perception throughout.

IMPRESSION: Left facial paralysis which appears to be chronic either secondary to a trauma in the past or residual from an old Bell palsy. A brainstem lesion, although unlikely, should be further investigated.

RECOMMENDATIONS: I have taken the liberty of ordering an MRI scan of the brain, EEG, and auditory brainstem evoked response to rule out the aforementioned possibilities.

Analysis: Review the medical record *Facial Paralysis* to answer the following questions.

1. Describe the patient's speech pattern.

2. What part of the patient's memory was severely impaired?

3. Why couldn't the doctor test the patient's cerebellar function?

4. How was the motor evaluation described?

5. What was the diagnosis?

Supplemental Medical Record Activity 14–3

Hydrocephalus

Terminology

Terms in the table come from the medical record *Hydrocephalus* that follows. Use a medical dictionary such as *Taber's Cyclopedic Medical Dictionary,* the appendices of *Systems,* 6th ed., or other resources to define each term. Then review pronunciations for each term and practice by reading the medical record aloud.

Term	Definition
burr hole bĕr	
cephalic end sĕ-FĂL-ĭk	
cm	
craniotome KRĀ-nē-ō-tōm	
dura DOO-ră	
galea GĀ-lē-ă	
H_2O	
hydrocephalus hī-drō-SĔF-ă-lŭs	
ICU	
lateral ventricle LĂT-ĕr-ăl VĔN-trĭ-kl	
parietal scalp pă-RĪ-ĕ-tăl SKĂLP	
ventriculoperitoneal shunt vĕn-trĭk-ū-lō-pĕr-ĭ-tō-NĒ-ăl SHŬNT	

HYDROCEPHALUS

PREOPERATIVE DIAGNOSIS: Hydrocephalus.

POSTOPERATIVE DIAGNOSIS: Hydrocephalus.

PROCEDURE PERFORMED: Ventriculoperitoneal shunt.

ANESTHESIA: General endotracheal.

PROCEDURE: Patient was brought to the operating room and anesthetized with general endotracheal anesthesia. He was placed in supine position with the head turned to the left. The right posterior scalp was shaved and prepped and draped in continuity with the right neck, chest, and abdomen. The skin was infiltrated with Xylocaine with epinephrine. A curved incision was made in the right parietal scalp. This was carried down to the skull and a scalp flap reflected forward. A craniotome was used to make a burr hole. The dura was coagulated and opened and a brain needle passed into the atrium of the lateral ventricle on the second attempt. Eight centimeters of ventricular catheter were threaded through this opening into the lateral ventricle. There was free flow of ventricular fluid. An incision was made into the abdomen and carried down through the anterior rectus sheath. The rectus abdominis muscle was separated and the posterior rectus sheath and peritoneum opened. The two incisions were connected with a shunt passer and kink-resistant peritoneal catheter threaded from the peritoneal end deep to the anterior rectus sheath through the shunt passer to the scalp. The peritoneum and posterior sheath were closed with 2-0 Vicryl. The cephalic end of the peritoneal catheter was attached to the shunt connector, which was attached to the distal end of a medium-pressure flat-bottom Mischler reservoir. The proximal end of the reservoir was attached to the right-angled connector which was connected to the ventricular end of the shunt tubing. All connections were ligated with 2-0 silk. The ventricular catheter was then obstructed, air flushed out of the shunt reservoir, and peritoneal tube and opening pressure measured. The opening pressure was 0.9 cm of H_2O. The ventricular catheter was again checked and there was free flow of ventricular fluid into the syringe. Four millimeters of preservative-free gentamicin were injected. The patient had been pretreated with antibiotics systemically and shunt hardware soaked in bacitracin. The 233 butterfly which had been used to puncture the proximal reservoir of the shunt was now removed. The galea was closed with

2-0 Vicryl and the skin with staples. A subcuticular layer of 4-0 Vicryl was placed and Steri-Strips placed on the skin. The patient was taken to the ICU with stable vital signs. Blood loss was trivial. The patient tolerated the procedure well.

Analysis: Review the medical record *Hydrocephalus* to answer the following questions.

1. What instrument was used to create the burr hole?

_____

2. Where was the brain needle positioned?

_____

3. What occurred when the ventricle was entered?

_____

4. What prophylactic treatment did the patient undergo?

_____

5. What type of suture did they use to close the galea?

_____

■ ■ ■ ■ Chapter 15–Special Senses

Supplemental Medical Record Activity 15–1

Chronic Suppurative Otitis Media

Terminology

Terms in the table come from the medical record *Chronic Suppurative Otitis Media* that follows. Use a medical dictionary such as *Taber's Cyclopedic Medical Dictionary,* the appendices of *Systems,* 6th ed., or other resources to define each term. Then review pronunciations for each term and practice by reading the medical record aloud.

Term	Definition
canaloplasty kă-NĂL-ō-plăs-tē	
cerumen sĕ-ROO-mĕn	
eustachian tube ū-STĀ-shĕn	
ossicular chain ŏ-SĬK-ū-lăr	
peritympanic incision pĕr-ĭ-tĭm-PĂN-ĭk ĭn-SĬ-zhŭn	
postauricular pōst-aw-RĬK-ū-lăr	
purulent debris PŪR-ū-lĕnt dĕ-BRĒ	
resected rē-SĔK-tĕd	
tympanic membrane perforation tĭm-PĂN-ĭk MĔM-brān pĕr-fō-RĀ-shŭn	
tympanosclerosis tĭm-pă-nō-sklĕ-RŌ-sĭs	

CHRONIC SUPPURATIVE OTITIS MEDIA

FINDINGS: This 14-year-old girl had a near-total tympanic membrane perforation. The small remnant of the tympanic membrane superiorly had tympanosclerosis present, so a total perforation was created.

MUCOSA: The middle ear mucosa was mildly inflamed. There was no active infection.

EUSTACHIAN TUBE: The eustachian tube was not visually obstructed. Furthermore, I was able to easily pass #00, #0, and #1 lacrimal probes without difficulty. A #2 lacrimal probe had too much tension to pass easily.

OSSICLES: I was concerned about her ossicular chain since the amount of hearing loss is more than I would usually anticipate with just a perforation alone. On close examination of the ossicular chain, the malleus was partially immobilized, but this improved considerably with removal of the tympanosclerosis surrounding the neck of the malleus and handle of the malleus. The incus long process was slightly eroded, but there was good continuity. The stapes was intact and mobile.

OPERATIVE DESCRIPTION: Patient was placed in the supine position on the operating table. General endotracheal anesthesia was administered. A small amount of hair was shaved from the postauricular region. The left ear was prepped and draped in the usual fashion.

The skin of the left ear canal was carefully cleaned of dead skin, cerumen, and hardened purulent debris. Using angled and straight Beaver blades, a posterior canal flap was incised and elevated from the bone of the external auditory canal.

CANALOPLASTY: A peritympanic incision was made. The tympanic membrane remnant was reflected inferiorly off the handle of the malleus. Diseased portions of the tympanic membrane and fibrosis at the perforation edge were resected using microscissors. Following placement of saline-soaked Gelfoam to support the graft, the grafts were placed underneath the medial canal skin and tympanic membrane remnant. Polysporin ointment was instilled into the ear canal.

Weitlaner retractors were removed. Hemostasis was obtained using electrocautery. The mastoid fascia was approximated using interrupted 3-0 Vicryl sutures. Wound care and dressings were carried out.

Patient was brought to the postanesthesia care unit in stable condition. There were no intraoperative complications. Blood loss was negligible.

FUTURE PLAN: The patient's conductive hearing loss will be reevaluated over the next 6 to 18 months to determine if there is any significant residual conductive loss. She will have to be followed to determine if tympanosclerosis will refix the ossicular chain.

Analysis: Review the medical record *Chronic Suppurative Otitis Media* to answer the following questions.

1. Why was tympanoplasty performed?

   _____

2. Was there an active infection?

   _____

3. How did the surgeon determine if the eustachian tube was obstructed?

   _____

4. What type of incision was made?

   _____

5. What type of suture did the surgeon use to close the mastoid fascia?

   _____

6. Examine Figure 15–3. Notice the location of the ossicles in relation to the tympanic membrane. Which ossicle is attached to the tympanic membrane?

   _____

7. What item was used to support the graft in the ear canal?

   _____

Supplemental Medical Record Activity 15–2

Cataract

Terminology

Terms in the table come from the medical record *Cataract* that follows. Use a medical dictionary such as *Taber's Cyclopedic Medical Dictionary*, the appendices of *Systems*, 6th ed., or other resources to define each term. Then review pronunciations for each term and practice by reading the medical record aloud.

Term	Definition
cataract KĂT-ă-răkt	
BP	
c/d ratio	
conjunctiva kŏn-jŭnk-TĪ-vă	
EOMs	
exudate ĔKS-ū-dāt	
foveal reflexes FŌ-vē-ăl RĔ-flĕks-ĕz	
gonioscopy gō-nē-ŎS-cō-pē	
iridodonesis ĭr-ĭd-ō-dō-NĒ-sĭs	
lacrimal apparatus LĂK-rĭm-ăl ăp-ă-RĂT-ŭs	
normocephalic nor-mō-sĕ-FĂL-ĭk	
PERRLA	
retinopathy rĕt-ĭn-ŎP-ă-thē	
sclerae SKLĔR-ē	
synechiae sĭ-NĔ-kē-ē	
trabecular meshwork tră-BĔK-ū-lăr MĔSH-wĕrk	
WD	
WN	

CATARACT

HISTORY

CHIEF COMPLAINT: Poor vision, left eye, slowly progressive apparently due to cataract. Vision can no longer be improved with new glasses or a pinhole. In addition, the patient's vision is markedly reduced in bright light and under night driving conditions. He has difficulty reading and driving an automobile due to glare symptoms from the left eye. The patient enters for cataract extraction with implantation of an intraocular lens, left eye, if possible. The risks, alternatives, and complications, to include blindness and death, have all been discussed, understood, and accepted. The patient has been cleared for the above surgery under local anesthesia by his primary care physician.

MEDICATIONS: Timoptic 0.5% each eye; Bleph-10 to lids, each eye four times a day; zinc sulfate, 50 mg twice a day after meals.

PHYSICAL EXAMINATION

PHYSICAL EXAM: WD, WN 83-year-old black male in no distress, looks stated age. BP 122/72.

HEAD: Normocephalic.

NECK: Supple, no adenopathy.

ENT: Clear.

EYES: Vision R = 20/80-2; L = 20/100+1 unimproved with a pinhole. Vision with the Brightness Acuity Tester in the left eye using low intensity is further reduced to 20/100-2; in medium intensity 20/200 and in high intensity to 20/400. Tension R = 16 mm; L = 16 mm Hg. PERRLA. EOMs full. Lids, lacrimal apparatus, conjunctivae, and sclerae clear in each eye.

Slit Lamp: Corneas and anterior chambers are clear in each eye and of average depth, with a 2 to 3+ nuclear and cortical cataract in situ; left eye worse than right. There is no iridodonesis.

Gonioscopy: Left eye: shows the angle wide open through the scleral spur 360 degrees with 2+ pigment in the trabecular meshwork. There is no peripheral anterior synechiae nor is there any angle recession.

Fundi: Left eye: hazy view due to cataract but with the binocular indirect ophthalmoscope grade II A-S changes are visible. Right eye: There is Grade II A-S retinopathy. There is no hemorrhage, exudate or retinal break visible in each eye. There are no foveal reflexes. The c/d ratio is 0.3:0.4 in each.

IMPRESSION:
1. Cataract, left eye worse than right, senile type.
2. Grade II A-S retinopathy in each eye.
3. Glaucoma, open angle, mild, well controlled.

Analysis: Review the medical record *Cataract* to answer the following questions.

1. What is causing poor vision in the left eye?

   _____

2. Did new glasses or pinhole improve the patient's vision?

   _____

3. When is the patient's vision the poorest?

   _____

4. Did the patient have any bleeding, exudates, or tears in the retinas?

   _____

5. What is the diagnosis regarding glaucoma?

   _____

Supplemental Medical Record Activities Answer Key

If you choose to have your students type and format the supplement at medical records in this Activity Pack, you can find correctly formatted versions in the instructional ancillaries section of http://davisplus.fadavis.com/gylys/systems/.

■ ■ ▪ Chapter 4–Body Structure

Supplemental Medical Record Activity 4–1

Radiology Report of the Skull, Facial Bones, and Orbits

Terminology

Term	Definition
anterior	Pertaining to or relating to the front or, in anatomical nomenclature, the ventral or abdominal side of the body
antrum ĂN-trŭm	Cavity or chamber that is nearly closed and usually surrounded by bone
AP	Anteroposterior
comminuted fracture KŎM-ĭ-nū-tĕd	Fracture in which the bone is broken or splintered into pieces
frontal sinus FRŬN-tăl SĪ-nŭs	Cavity located in the frontal bone of the skull
lateral LĂT-ĕr-ăl	Pertaining to the side
mandible MĂN-dĭ-bl	Lower jaw bone
oblique ō-BLĒK	Referring to a 45-degree angle
opaque ō-PĀK	Unable to be penetrated by light rays from the x-ray
PA	Posteroanterior
zygoma zī-GŌ-mă	Long arch that joins zygomatic processes of the temporal and malar bones on the sides of the skull

Analysis:

1. What four body structures were x-rayed?

   Skull, mandible, zygoma, sinuses, and orbits

2. What views were included in the skull series?

   Standard skull series with lateral, PA, and Towne views; AP views of the mandible, base views of the zygoma, Waters view of the sinuses, and Reese views of the orbits

3. What is a comminuted fracture?

   A broken bone that has splintered into pieces.

4. How did the physician come to the conclusion that the zygoma was fractured in its central portion?

   The left zygoma was not seen on the base view except in the anterior and posterior portions, suggesting that it was fractured in its central portion with some depression.

Supplemental Medical Record Activity 4–2

Gunshot Wound to the Chest

Terminology

Term	Definition
cannulate KĂN-ū-lāt	To insert a tube into a duct or cavity
comatose KŌ-mă-tōs	State of unconsciousness
contused kŏn-TOOZD	Bruised
diaphoretic dī-ă-fō-RĔT-ĭk	Excessive perspiration
diaphragm DĪ-ă-frăm	Major muscle of respiration, separating the thoracic and abdominal cavities
inferior vena cava VĒ-nă KĀ-vă	Vein that carries the blood to the heart from the lower extremities and trunk of the body
intercostal space ĭn-tĕr-KŎS-tăl	Area between the ribs
pericardial sac pĕr-ĭ-KĂR-dē-ăl	Membrane which surrounds the heart
pericardial tamponade pĕr-ĭ-KĂR-dē-ăl tăm-pŏn-ĀD	Acute compression of the heart due to collection of the blood in the sac surrounding the heart
posterolateral pŏs-tĕr-ō-LĂT-ĕr-ăl	Pertaining to the back and side of the body or any structure
right quadrant KWŎD-rănt	Right-upper fourth of the abdomen
sternum STĔR-nŭm	Breast bone
superior vena cava VĒ-nă KĀ-vă	Vein that carries the blood to the heart from the upper extremities, head, neck, and chest
ventricle VĔN-trĭk-l	One of the two lower chambers of the heart that forces blood out of the heart into the arteries

Analysis:

1. Where did the bullet enter the patient's body?

   The bullet entered the left chest at approximately the fifth intercostal space, just to the left of the sternum.

2. What direction did the bullet travel through the body?

   The trajectory was right-to-left on an axis pointing from the anterior right chest to the posterior left flank.

3. Where does the bullet appear to be lodged?

   In the left posterior back

4. Was the diaphragm injured?

   No, it was not violated.

5. How did the physician stop the active bleeding of the heart?

   By placing a finger over the hole and suturing the heart closed over Teflon pledgets

■ ■ ■ Chapter 5–Integumentary System

Supplemental Medical Record Activity 5–1

Pigmented Solar Keratosis

Terminology

Term	Definition
cherry angioma ăn-jē-Ō-mă	Bright red tumor made up of blood vessels that occurs most commonly in older individuals
excoriated acne ĕks-KŌ-rē-ă-tĭd ĂK-nē	Inflammatory skin disease of the sebaceous glands caused by squeezing the pustules and comedos (blackheads)
idiopathic guttate hypomelanosis ĭd-ē-ō-PĂTH-ĭk GOO-tāt hī-pō-mĕl-ă-NŌ-sĭs	Depigmented, irregular blotches on the skin, usually affecting the shins of adults
photoprotection fō-tō-prō-TĔK-shŭn	Any protective substance or clothing used to keep sun rays from damaging the skin
pigmented solar keratosis PĬG-mĕnt-ĕd SŌ-lăr kĕr-ă-TŌ-sĭs	Horny growth, such as a wart or callus, that changes color due to the sun
seborrheic keratosis sĕb-ō-RĒ-ĭk kĕr-ă-TŌ-sĭs	Benign, noninvasive tumor of epidermal origin developing in the form of numerous yellow or brown raised lesions

Analysis:

1. What was the predisposing factor causing the patient's present condition?

   Exposing her skin to the sun

2. What did the doctor recommend to the patient to prevent future problems with solar keratosis?

   Protect her skin from the sun (phot-protection)

3. What treatment was performed on the precancerous lesions?

   Freezing the lesions with liquid nitrogen on an applicator

4. When does the doctor want to see the patient again?

   Only as required

Supplemental Medical Record Activity 5–2

Severe Pressure Ulcer, Left Foot, Now Gangrenous

Terminology

Term	Definition
AK	Above the knee
amputation ăm-pū-TĀ-shŭn	Cut off or remove an extremity
arteriosclerosis ăr-tē-rē-ō-sklĕ-RŌ-sĭs	Hardening of the arteries, causing poor circulation
contractures kŏn-TRĂK-chŭrz	Shortening of the distance between two points, resulting in the patient being unable to straighten an extremity
debridement dā-brĕd-MŎN	Removal of devitalized tissue
flexion FLĔK-shŭn	Bending
gangrenous GĂNG-grĕn-ŭs	Necrotic condition caused by a decrease in blood supply to an area
pressure ulcer	Chronic ulceration that appears on pressure spots due to confinement to a bed or wheelchair for long periods of time; also called *decubitus ulcer*

Analysis:

1. What measures did the health care providers initially use to lessen the problems caused by heel pressure?

   <u>*Local care, debridement, physical therapy, and good padding*</u>

2. Why was it difficult for the patient to keep pressure off the heel?

   <u>*Because of the patient's severe senile mental state and acquired flexion contractures of the lower extremities*</u>

3. What type of contractures did the physician identify?

   <u>*Flexion*</u>

4. Was the right foot as bad as the left?

   <u>*No, there was a smaller pressure ulcer on the right heel but the remainder of the right foot was in good condition.*</u>

5. What type of amputation did the doctor perform?

   <u>*Above the knee*</u>

■ ■ ■ **Chapter 6–Digestive System**

Supplemental Medical Record Activity 6–1

Esophagogastroduodenoscopy (EGD) with Biopsy

Terminology

Term	Definition
antral ĂN-trăl	Pertaining to a chamber or cavity
EGD	Esophagogastroduodenoscopy
endoscopy ĕn-DŎS-kō-pē	Procedure using an instrument that visualizes an interior structure of the body
epigastric ĕp-ĭ-GĂS-trĭk	Relating to the region above the stomach
erythematous ĕr-ĭ-THĔM-ă-tŭs	Pertaining to or marked by diffuse redness
esophagitis ē-sŏf-ă-JĪ-tĭs	Inflammation of the esophagus
esophagoscope ē-SŎF-ă-gō-skōp	Instrument to examine the esophagus
fundus FŬN-dŭs	Base or bottom part of a hollow organ
Helicobacter hĕl-ĭ-kō-BĂK-tĕr	Bacterial organism associated with gastric and peptic ulcers as well as gastric cancers
IV	Intravenous
mg	Milligram (1/1,000 of a gram)
oropharynx or-ō-FĂR-ĭnks	Part of the pharynx lying between the soft palate and the upper portion of the epiglottis
retroflex RĔ-trō-flĕks	Bend backward
squamocolumnar junction skwā-mō-kō-LŬM-năr JŬNK-shŭn	Point in the cervical canal where the squamous and columnar epithelia meet
ulceration ŭl-sĕr-Ā-shŭn	Suppuration occurring on a free surface such as the skin and mucous membrane

Analysis:

1. What anesthetic was administered for this procedure?

   Cetacaine spray. Demerol 50 mg. Versed 4 mg IV

2. What type of endoscope was used for the procedure?

   Pentax video upper endoscope

3. How far was the endoscope placed in the GI tract?

   As far as the third portion of the duodenum

4. Why was a biopsy performed?

   To test for Helicobacter

5. Were ulcers found in the mucosa?

No

6. What was the final diagnosis?

Mild antral gastritis and distal esophagitis

Supplemental Medical Record Activity 6–2

Fissure-in-Ano

Terminology

Term	Definition
defecation dĕf-ĕ-KĀ-shŭn	Evacuation of fecal material from the bowel
epidural anesthesia ĕp-ĭ-DOO-răl ăn-ĕs-THĒ-zē-ă	Anesthetic injected between the vertebral spines into the extradural space
excision ĕk-SĬ-zhŭn	Surgical removal (cutting out)
external hemorrhoids HĔM-ō-roydz	Varicose dilatations situated distal to the pectinate line and covered with anal skin
fissure-in-ano FĬSH-ūr ĭn-Ā-nō	Linear ulcer (groove) at the margin of the anus
fissurectomy fĭsh-ūr-ĔK-tō-mē	Excision (surgical removal) of a fissure
hemogram HĒ-mō-grăm	Record or graphic representation of a complete blood count; also called *peripheral blood picture*
internal hemorrhoids HĔM-ō-roydz	Varicose dilatation above the pectinate line covered with mucous membrane
microscopic mī-krō-SKŎ-pĭc	Pertaining to something extremely small in size and requiring the use of a microscope for visualization
morbid obesity MOR-bĭd ō-BĒ-sĭ-tē	Body mass index (BMI) of 40 or greater, which is generally 100 or more pounds over ideal body weight.
sentinel pile SĔN-tĭn-ĕl PĪ-ĕl	Hemorrhoidlike thickening of the mucous membrane at the lower end of an anal fissure
urinalysis ū-rĭ-NĂL-ĭ-sĭs	Examination of urine

Analysis:

1. How long had this patient been having pain?

   Two months

2. What word in this report is synonymous with pile?

   Hemorrhoid

3. In what part of the anus was the fissure located?

   Posterior area

4. How is morbid obesity defined?

   When the patient has a body mass index (BMI) of 40 or greater, which is generally 100 or more pounds over ideal body weight.

5. What did the doctor do to the patient's anal area following excision of the fissure?

   Dilated the anal canal

Supplemental Medical Record Activity 6–3

Inguinal Hernia

Terminology

Term	Definition
bilaterally bī-LĂT-ĕr-ăl-lē	On both sides
hernia HĔR-nē-ă	Protrusion of an organ or structure through an anatomical wall
hesitancy HĔS-ĭ-tĕn-sē	Inability to start the urinary stream
inguinal ĬNG-gwĭ-năl	Pertaining to the region of the groin
laparoscopic lăp-ă-rō-SKŎP-ĭK	Pertaining to an endoscope designed to permit visual examination of the abdominal cavity
micturition mĭk-tū-RĬ-shŭn	Urination
prostatitis prŏs-tă-TĪ-tĭs	Inflammation of the prostate
testes TĔS-tēs	Structures responsible for the production of sperm
umbilicus ŭm-BĬL-ĭ-kŭs	Navel
varicocele VĂR-ĭ-kō-sēl	Swelling of the veins of the spermatic cord

Analysis:

1. How did the patient discover he had a hernia?

   He had incidental notice of the hernia during a physical examination.

2. What two symptoms did the patient experience?

   Increased fullness and an occasional heavy sensation in the left groin

3. How was the urination of the patient described?

   Difficulty initiating micturition with urinary hesitancy and occasional frequency.

4. Which two treatments were described to repair the hernia?

   Conventional versus laparoscopic repair

5. Which method of repair did the physician recommend?

   Laparoscopic repair

■ ■ ■ **Chapter 7–Respiratory System**

Supplemental Medical Record Activity 7–1

Asthma (Child)

Terminology

Term	Definition
aerosolized ĔR-ō-sō-līzd	Solution or drug that is presented in a fine mist
albuterol ăl-BŪ-tĕr-ăl	Bronchodilator that causes bronchial muscles to relax, thereby expanding air passages and resulting in increased air flow
asthma ĂZ-mă	Condition marked by sudden involuntary shortness of breath due to spasmodic contractions of the bronchi
expiratory wheeze ĕks-PĪ-ră-tor-ē HWĒZ	Whistling sound made when exhaling
organomegaly or-gă-nō-MĔG-ă-lē	Enlargement of internal body organs
ventilated VĔN-tĭ-lā-tĕd	Exchange of air carried out mechanically using positive pressure breathing apparatus

Analysis:

1. How long has this child had a history of asthma?

   Since birth

2. Why was the child returned to Pope Memorial Hospital after being treated earlier at Travis Medical Facility?

   Because his chest was tight and he had difficulty breathing even after being treated with bronchodilators

3. What medication did the child receive in the emergency department?

   He received 30 mg of prednisone orally.

4. What contributory factors might be significant for this child's illness?

   Family history of asthma on mother's side

5. What type of lung sounds were heard upon examination?

   Breath sounds clear bilaterally with somewhat decreased air exchange and diffuse expiratory wheeze. Work of breathing is mildly to moderately increased.

Supplemental Medical Record Activity 7–2

Bronchoscopy

Terminology

Term	Definition
biopsies BĪ-ŏp-sēz	Surgical removal of samplings of tissue for diagnostic purposes
bronchoscope BRŎNG-kŏ-skōp	Lighted, lensed instrument used for viewing the interior surface of the bronchi
bronchoscopy brŏng-KŎS-kŏ-pē	Process of visually examining the bronchi
brushings BRŬSH-ĭngz	Samples of tissue taken by sweeping or gently rubbing a fine brushlike tip against the tissue
carina kă-RĪ-nă	Ridgelike structure that runs from front to back between the openings of the two bronchi
endotracheal lesion ĕn-dō-TRĀ-kē-ăl LĒ-zhŭn	Growth within the trachea
epiglottis ĕp-ĭ-GLŎT-ĭs	Leaf-shaped flap that closes over the larynx while swallowing
infiltration ĭn-fĭl-TRĀ-shŭn	Process of entering the tissue spaces
mass	Generic term for lesion or tumor
medially MĒ-dē-ăl-lē	Toward the middle
mg	Milligram (1/1,000 of a gram)
mL	Milliliter (1/1,000 of a liter)
nasotracheal tube nā-zō-TRĀ-kē-ăl	Tube designed specifically to enter through the opening of the nose and extend to the beginning of the trachea
occluded ō-KLŪ-dĭd	Obstructed; closed off
saturation săt-ū-RĀ-shŭn	Condition of being saturated; when a substance cannot absorb or hold any more solution

Analysis:

1. Refer to Figure 7–1 to locate the trachea and bronchi. How far was the bronchoscope inserted?

   Right upper lobe, right lower lobe, and right middle lobe and into the left lower lobe bronchus

2. What was the color of the secretions in the right lower lobe of the lung?

   Whitish

3. What was the finding regarding the right lung?

   No endobronchial lesion or external bronchial compression

4. In which part of the left lung was the mass identified?

   Middle to lower section of the upper lung

5. What was obtained from the left mainstem bronchus tumor?

   Multiple biopsies, washings, and brushings

Supplemental Medical Record Activity 7–3

Peritonsillar Abscess

Terminology

Term	Definition
cervical adenopathy SĔR-vǐ-kăl ăd-ĕ-NŎP-ă-thē	Disease process of the cervical glands
edema ĕ-DĒ-mă	Excessive accumulation of fluid in tissue
erythema ĕr-ĭ-THĒ-mă	Redness
erythematous ĕr-ĭ-THĔM-ă-tŭs	Pertaining to redness
mucopurulent mū-kō-PŪR-ū-lĕnt	Thick, puslike mucous discharge
nasopharyngitis nā-zō-făr-ĭn-JĪ-tĭs	Inflammation of the nose and throat
oropharynx or-ō-FĂR-ĭnks	Back of the throat
peritonsillar abscess pĕr-ĭ-TŎN-sĭ-lărĂB-sĕs	Infected wound surrounding the tonsils
pharyngitis făr-ĭn-JĪ-tĭs	Inflammation of the throat
purulent PŪR-ū-lĕnt	Containing pus
rhinoscopy rī-NŎS-kō-pē	Procedure to visually examine the nose
submandibular sŭb-măn-DĬB-ū-lăr	Below the mandible (lower jaw bone)
tonsillectomy tŏn-sĭl-ĔK-tō-mē	Excision of the tonsils

Analysis:

1. What type of recurrent illness was identified in the patient's medical history?

   Recurrent pharyngitis and peritonsillar abscess

2. Where was the noticeable swelling?

   Left submandibular lymph node

3. What did the nasopharyngeal examination show?

   Mucopurulent drainage with erythematous inflammation of the adenoid pad

4. Was the drainage the same inside the nose?

   No, there was no purulent drainage.

5. What was the immediate treatment?

   Augmentin and ibuprofen

Supplemental Medical Record Activity 7–4

Allergic Rhinitis

Terminology

Term	Definition
exacerbates ĕks-ĂS-ĕr-bātz	Increases in severity
hypertrophy hī-PĔR-trŏ-fē	Increase in the size of the body, an organ, or a structure due to growth rather than tumor formation
nasopharynx nā-zō-FĂR-ĭnks	Part of the pharynx situated above the soft palate
otoscopic ō-tō-SKŎP-ĭk	Pertaining to an instrument used to examine the ear
rhinitis rī-NĪ-tĭs	Inflammation of the nasal mucosa
rhinorrhea rī-nō-RĒ-ă	Thin, watery discharge from the nose
septoplasty SĔP-tō-plăs-tē	Repair of the nasal septum
turbinate TŬR-bĭn-āt	Shaped like an inverted cone

Analysis:

1. What surgeries did the patient have last year?

   Septoplasty and turbinate reduction

2. What was the outcome of last year's surgery?

   Significant improvement in airway passage

3. What seasonal symptoms are currently noted by the patient?

   Sneezing and watery rhinorrhea as well as a tickling of the palate and burning of the eyes

4. How is the nasal mucosa described?

   Somewhat pale and edematous with a serous discharge

5. What was the recommendation of the physician?

   Double-strength Vancenase AQ and Allegra; see an allergist to undergo definitive allergy testing.

■ ■ ■ **Chapter 8–Cardiovascular System**

Supplemental Medical Record Activity 8–1

Cardiomyopathy and Supraventricular Arrhythmias

Terminology

Term	Definition
angiography ăn-jē-ŎG-ră-fē	Invasive radiological procedure to evaluate pressure in the arteries and determine cardiac output
arrhythmias ă-RĬTH-mē-ă	Any deviations from the normal pattern of a heartbeat.
atherosclerosis ăth-ĕr-ō-sklĕ-RŌ-sĭs	Hardening of the arteries
bradyarrhythmias brăd-ē-ă-RĬTH-mē-ăz	Heartbeat less than 60 beats per minute associated with an irregular heart rhythm
bundle branch block	Blockage of the conduction system on one of the branches of the bundle of His
cardiomegaly kăr-dē-ō-MĔG-ă-lē	Enlargement of the heart
claudication klaw-dĭ-KĀ-shŭn	Complex of symptoms that occurs when walking and ceases when walking stops; also called *lameness*
diaphoresis dī-ă-fō-RĒ-sĭs	Excessive perspiration
differential dĭf-ĕr-ĔN-shăl	Hematological identification of the various types of white blood cells
echocardiography ĕk-ō-kăr-dē-ŎG-ră-fē	Imaging technique that uses ultrasound to assess the structures of the heart
embolus ĔM-bō-lŭs	Clot
fibrillation fĭ-brĭl-Ā-shŭn	Irregular, random contraction of heart fibers
hypercholesterolemia hī-pĕr-kō-lĕs-tĕr-ŏl-Ē-mē-ă	Excessive levels of cholesterol in the blood
hypertension hī-pĕr-TĔN-shŭn	Increase in the amount of pressure (tension) in the blood vessels
icterus ĬK-tĕr-ŭs	Jaundice (yellow-orange discoloration)
palpitations păl-pĭ-TĀ-shŭnz	Rapid or irregular heart beat
petechiae pē-TĒ-kē-ē	Small, pinpoint hemorrhages
PMI	Point of maximal impulse
PT	Prothrombin time; physical therapy

Term	Definition
PTT	Partial thromboplastin time (more sensitive than PT in evaluating the adequacy of fibrin clot formation and also measures intrinsic factors)
syncope SĬN-kō-pē	Fainting
transient ischemic attack TRĂN-sē-ĕnt ĭs-KĒ-mĭk ă-TĂK	Brief episodes of decrease in blood supply to vascular areas

Analysis:

1. Why was Mr. Mayfield treated with digoxin following his evaluation at Presbyterian Hospital?

   To control the atrial fibrillation

2. What was the probable cause of the episode of rapid atrial fibrillation when Mr. Mayfield was first seen at El Camino Hospital?

   Systemic embolus to his abdomen

3. Refer to Figure 8-2. Notice the location of the aorta and the aortic semilunar valve. What procedure did Dr. Robert Terhune perform?

   Composite replacement of the aortic valve and aortic root

4. Why was the patient admitted following his examination in the emergency department?

   To observe him and do further workup regarding the cause of his presyncopal episodes

5. What family history, if any, may have contributed to the patient's problems?

   Atherosclerosis

6. What tests will Dr. Munier perform?

   Electrophysiological testing; possible tilt table testing to rule out vasovagal episodes and significant ventricular arrhythmias

Supplemental Medical Record Activity 8–2

Coronary Artery Disease with Myocardial Infarction

Terminology

Term	Definition
bypass graft surgery BĬ-păs GRĂFT SŬR-jĕr-ē	Surgical correction in which a graft is sutured above and below the area of blockage in the coronary artery
coronary angiography KOR-ō-nă-rē ăn-jē-ŎG-ră-fē	Invasive radiological procedure that involves feeding catheters through the arterial system into the heart and injecting radiopaque dye to determine the status of the coronary arteries
CPK	Creatinine phosphokinase (enzyme released into the bloodstream after a myocardial infarction)
ischemic cardiomyopathy ĭs-KĒ-mĭk kăr-dē-ō-mī-ŎP-ă-thē	Disease of the heart muscle caused by lack of adequate blood supply
laparotomy lăp-ăr-ŎT-ō-mē	Procedure used to cut into the abdomen
myocardial infarction mī-ō-KĂR-dē-ăl ĭn-FĂRK-shŭn	Tissue death caused by occlusion of a blood vessel in the heart muscle

Term	Definition
occlusion ō-CLOO-shŭn	Blockage
stenosis stĕ-NŌ-sĭs	Narrowing
ventricular and supraventricular arrhythmias vĕn-TRĬK-ū-lăr, soo-pră-vĕn-TRĬK-ū-lăr ă-RĬTH-mē-ăz	Irregular rhythm of the lower and upper chambers of the heart

Analysis:

1. What diagnosis was made at Crescent City Hospital?

    Myocardial infarction

2. Why was the patient readmitted?

    Heart failure and cardiac arrhythmias

3. What information did the cardiac catheterization provide?

    Ejection fraction around 30% to 35% and severe left main coronary artery stenosis and right coronary artery occlusion

4. To what extent are the carotids blocked?

    60% to 70%

5. What is his anticipated life expectancy based on his history of cancer?

    Two to 3 years

6. What procedure will be performed?

    Coronary artery bypass graft

■ ■ ■ Chapter 9–Blood, Lymph, and Immune Systems

Supplemental Medical Record Activity 9–1

Bone Marrow Study Following Chemotherapy

Terminology

Term	Definition
basophilic bā-sō-FĬL-ĭk	Pertaining to the type of granulocyte that stains with a basic or alkaline dye
CBC	Complete blood count
G-CSF	Granulocyte colony-stimulating factor
intraoperative radiotherapy ĭn-tră-ŎP-ĕr-ă-tĭv rā-dē-ō-THĔR-ă-pē	Treatment using radioisotopes that are applied directly to the operative site while the cavity is exposed
leukocytosis loo-kō-sī-TŌ-sĭs	Increase in white blood cells in the blood

Term	Definition
myelosuppression mĭ-ĕ-lō-sŭ-PRĔSH-ŭn	Inhibition of bone marrow activity
neuroblastoma nū-rō-blăs-TŌ-mă	Malignant tumor originating in the nervous system
occult ŏ-KŬLT	Hidden
orthochromatophilic or-thō-krō-măt-ō-FĬL-ĭk	Normally colored or stained
polychromatophilic pŏl-ē-krō-măt-ō-FĬL-ĭk	Capable of staining with many colors
segs	Segmented neutrophils

Analysis:

1. What procedures were previously performed on the patient?

   Several laparotomies and one course of intraoperative radiotherapy

2. Why was a bone marrow aspirate performed on the patient?

   To rule out the appearance of any occult neuroblastoma in his bone marrow

3. What appears to have caused the patient's leukocytosis?

   G-CSF, which stimulates the production of granulocytes

4. What was the result of the Wright stain bone marrow study?

   It failed to reveal any obvious neuroblastoma rosettes or tumor clumps.

5. Why was a sample of heparinized bone marrow sent to Dr. Seeger's laboratory?

   For monoclonal antibody assessment for occult neuroblastoma

Supplemental Medical Record Activity 9–2

Stage III-A Hodgkin Disease

Terminology

Term	Definition
Hodgkin disease HŎJ-kĭn dĭ-ZĒZ	Malignant disease of the lymph system that primarily affects lymph nodes
megakaryocytes mĕg-ă-KĂR-ē-ō-sīt	Blood cells with large nuclei
monos MŎN-ōs	Monocytes

Term	Definition
morphological examination mor-fō-LŎJ-ĭk-kāl	Microscopic examination used to study the shapes of blood cells
neutropenia noo-trō-PĒ-nē-ă	Deficiency of neutrophils
segs SĔGZ	Segmented neutrophils
spicules SPĬK-ūlz	Sharp, needlelike forms
thrombocytopenia thrŏm-bō-sī-tō-PĒ-nē-ă	Deficiency of platelets (thrombocytes)

Analysis:

1. Why was a bone marrow examination performed on this patient?

   To rule out bone marrow involvement with her Hodgkin disease

2. What was noted in the peripheral blood regarding platelets?

   Platelets are 160,000 (increased from 44,000 2 days earlier).

3. In the bone marrow aspirate, what was the predominant cell observed?

   Myeloid

4. What was the impression regarding malignancy?

   No evidence of malignant disease

■ ■ ■ Chapter 10–Musculoskeletal System

Supplemental Medical Record Activity 10–1

Spinal Stenosis

Terminology

Term	Definition
concentric annular disk bulge kŏn-SĔN-trĭk ĂN-ū-lăr DĬSK	Ringlike protrusion of the intervertebral disk from the center outward
conus medullaris KŌ-nŭs mĕd-ū-LĂR-ĭs	Cone-shaped end of the spinal cord
facet arthropathy FĂS-ĕt ăr-THRŎP-ă-thē	Disease process of the vertebra where it articulates with another structure
intervertebral disk degeneration ĭn-tĕr-VĔRT-ĕ-brĕl DĬSK dē-gĕn-ĕr-Ā-shŭn	Breakdown of the fibrocartilage between the vertebral bodies of the spine
L2	Second lumbar vertebra

Term	Definition
MRI	Magnetic resonance imaging
osteophyte ŎS-tē-ō-fīt	Bony outgrowth
paraspinous pără-SPĪ-nŭs	Beside the spine
spinal stenosis SPĪ-năl stě-NŌ-sĭs	Narrowing of the openings in the spine
T1	First thoracic vertebra
thecal sac THĒ-kăl SĂK	Dura mater of the spinal cord

Analysis:

1. Why was this patient referred to x-ray?

   Low back and right leg pain

2. What kind of thecal sac flattening was evident in the L2 to L3 vertebral view?

   Mild ventral (belly side) flattening

3. At what levels was intervertebral disk degeneration noted?

   L4 to S1

4. What did the MRI reveal at L5 to S1?

   There is intervertebral disk degeneration.

5. Where is the conus medullaris located?

   At the level of the upper part of the lumbar vertebrae

Supplemental Medical Record Activity 10–2

Neck and Shoulder Pain Due to Auto Accident

Terminology

Term	Definition
C4	Fourth cervical vertebra
craniotomy krā-nē-ŎT-ō-mē	Incision in the skull
degenerative disk disease dē-GĚN-ĕr-ă-tĭv DĬSK	Breakdown of the fibrocartilage between the vertebrae
exacerbation ĕks-ăs-ĕr-BĀ-shŭn	Increase in the severity of a disease or disorder as marked by greater intensity in the patient's signs or symptoms
L5	Fifth lumbar vertebra
modalities mō-DĂL-ĭ-tēz	Forms of therapy

Term	Definition
physical therapy FĬZ-ĭ-kăl THĔR-ă-pē	Use of various modalities, such as heat, ice, water, massage, exercise, and ultrasound, to rehabilitate and restore normal body function after an injury or illness
S1	First sacral vertebra

Analysis:

1. Was the motor vehicle accident the primary cause of the patient's neck pain?

   No, her symptomatology was due to cancer.

2. What types of surgery did the patient have as a result of the cancer?

   Radical neck resection with pectoralis transfer as well as craniotomy, excision of bone fragment, abscess formation, and eye surgery

3. Why is it difficult for the physician to evaluate the patient's present condition?

   Because she has missed her appointments

4. What was the status of the patient's neck mobility prior to the motor vehicle accident?

   Marginal strength and mobility due to her neck cancer

Supplemental Medical Record Activity 10–3

Chronic Tendinitis

Terminology

Term	Definition
capitellum kăp-ĭ-TĔL-ŭm	Round eminence at lower end of the humerus that articulates with the radius
chondromalacia kŏn-drō-măl-Ā-shē-ă	Softening of cartilage
condylar KŎN-dĭ-lăr	Pertaining to a condyle (rounded protuberance at the end of a bone that forms an articulation)
dissection dĭ-SĔK-shŭn	Cutting parts to separate and study them
exsanguinating ĕks-SĂNG-gwĭn-ā-tĭng	Removing blood
hemostasis hē-mō-STĀ-sĭs	Arrest or control of bleeding
oblique ō-BLĔK	Slanting, diagonal
phlebitis flĕ-BĪ-tĭs	Inflammation of a vein
prophylactic prō-fĭ-LĂK-tĭk	Agent or regimen that contributes to the prevention of infection or disease
purulent PŬR-ū-lĕnt	Forming or containing pus; also called *suppurative*

Term	Definition
recalcitrant rē-CĂL-sĭ-trănt	Obstinate or unrelenting
supracondylar soo-pră-KŎN-dĭ-lăr	Relating to the area above a condyle
tendinitis tĕn-dĭn-Ī-tĭs	Inflammation of a tendon
tourniquet TOOR-nĭ-kĕt	Constrictor used on an extremity over an artery to control bleeding

Analysis:

1. How was the tendinitis described?

   As recalcitrant

2. What conservative treatment had the patient undergone prior to surgery?

   Corticosteroid injections, physical therapy, exercises, anti-inflammatory, and elbow sleeve

3. What complications were described to the patient?

   Infection; phlebitis; neurovascular tendon injury; anesthetic complications; failure of the procedure; recurrence, inadequate result; anesthetic problems; and others

4. After the arm was scrubbed and draped, what procedure was undertaken?

   The arm was exsanguinated.

5. What was the finding after incision?

   Typical chronic tendinitis

6. How was the synovial fluid described?

   As straw-colored and not purulent

■ ■ ■ **Chapter 11–Genitourinary System**

Supplemental Medical Record Activity 11–1

Testicular Mass

Terminology

Term	Definition
alpha-fetoprotein ĂL-fă FĒ-tō-prō-tēn	Plasma protein found in some embryonic tissue and in the blood of patients with tumors
anorexia ăn-ō-RĔK-sē-ă	Loss of appetite
epididymis ĕp-ĭ-DĬD-ĭ-mĭs	Structure that lies over the testes and stores sperm
fluctuance FLŬK-chū-ănts	Wavelike motion on palpation when fluid is present
GU	Genitourinary

Term	Definition
HCG	Human chorionic gonadotropin
hydrocele HĪ-drō-sēl	Collection of fluid in the testes
inhomogeneous ĭn-hō-mō-JĒ-nē-ŭs	Lacking composition of similar elements or structures
malaise mă-LĀZ	General body discomfort
mg	Milligram (1/1,000 of a gram)
phallus FĂL-ŭs	Penis
urethral ū-RĒ-thrăl	Pertaining to the urethra
voiding VOY-dĭng	Urinating

Analysis:

1. What were the patient's initial symptoms?

   Right testicular pain radiating to his right groin and right flank

2. What was the patient initially treated for?

   Infection of the epididymis

3. Did the patient have a urethral discharge?

   No

4. What did the scrotal ultrasound reveal?

   An inhomogeneous right testicular mass

5. What type of surgery is planned for the patient?

   Right inguinal exploration with possible radical orchiectomy

Supplemental Medical Record Activity 11–2

Monilial-type balanitis

Terminology

Term	Definition
Accu-Chek ĂK-ū-chĕk	Instrument that analyzes a drop of capillary blood to determine blood sugar level
chlamydia klă-MĬD-ē-ă	Sexually transmitted disease caused by the bacterium *Chlamydia trachomatis*
cultures KŬL-chŭrz	Propagation of microorganisms
dysuria dīs-Ū-rē-ă	Painful urination

Term	Definition
foreskin FOR-skĭn	Fold of skin that covers the glans penis; also called *prepuce*
frequency FRĒ-qwĕn-cē	Urinating at short intervals
GC	Gonorrhea
herpes HĔR-pēz	Sexually transmitted disease caused by the herpes virus
hypoglycemic agents hī-pō-glī-SĒ-mĭk Ā-jĕnts	Medications used to lower blood glucose level
monilial-type balanitis mō-NĬL-ē-ăl bă-lă-NĪ-tĭs	Inflammation of the glans penis caused by a yeast infection
uncircumcised ŭn-SĔR-kŭm-sĭzd	Condition in which the foreskin remains intact rather than being surgically removed
urgency ĔR-jĕn-sē	Sudden, compelling urge to urinate

Analysis:

1. What prompted the patient to seek medical care?

   The skin on his penis was peeling

2. Did the patient have any urinary problems?

   No

3. Was the patient taking medications for his glucose intolerance?

   Not presently because he depleted his oral hypoglycemics

4. Why did the doctor order cultures?

   To check for sexually transmitted diseases, specifically, gonorrhea, chlamydia, and herpes

■ ■ ■ **Chapter 12–Female Reproductive System**

Supplemental Medical Record Activity 12–1

Intrauterine Pregnancy

Terminology

Term	Definition
ab	Abortion
amnionitis ăm-nē-ō-NĪ-tĭs	Inflammation of the amnion
cesarean section sē-SĀR-ē-ăn SĔK-shŭn	Incision made through the abdominal and uterine walls to deliver a fetus

Term	Definition
effaced ĕ-FĀST	Situation in which the cervix is completely changed with only the thin external os remaining
footling breech FOOT-lĭng BRĒCH	Situation in which the foot or feet of the fetus present first
gestation jĕs-TĀ-shŭn	Length of time from conception to birth
gravida GRĂV-ĭ-dă	Woman who is pregnant
para PĂR-ă	Woman who has given birth to one or more viable infants
spontaneous abortion spŏn-TĀ-nē-ŭs ă-BOR-shŭn	Premature expulsion of the fetus that occurs naturally rather than by a medical procedure

Analysis:

1. What happened to this patient on November 9?

   She experienced spontaneous premature rupture of membranes.

2. Was the patient at term when labor started?

   No. She was only 31 to 32 weeks into her pregnancy.

3. What was the indication for cesarean section?

   The fetus is presenting in a footling breech position.

4. How many times was the patient pregnant?

   This is her third pregnancy.

Supplemental Medical Record Activity 12–2

Labor Examination in Adolescent Mother

Terminology

Term	Definition
anemic ă-NĒ-mĭk	Reduction in red blood cells
effaced ĕ-FĀST	Situation in which the cervix is changed to the point where it is flattened and the thin external os remains
gestation jĕs-TĀ-shŭn	Period from fertilization of the ovum until birth
ischial spines ĬS-kē-ăl	Bony prominence coming off the ischium
primigravida prī-mĭ-GRĂV-ĭ-dă	Woman who is pregnant for the first time; also called *gravida 1*
promontory PRŎM-ŏn-tōr-ē	Projection on the anterior border of the first sacral vertebra
vertex VĔR-tĕks	Top of a structure or organ

Analysis:

1. Why was the patient admitted to the hospital?

   Her bag of waters *spontaneously broke.*

2. What is the patient doing for her anemia?

   Taking oral iron three times daily

3. Does the doctor feel the patient will be able to have a vaginal delivery?

   No, there is a definite risk of the fetus not passing the midplane of the pelvis.

■ ■ ■ Chapter 13–Endocrine System

Supplemental Medical Record Activity 13–1

Primary Hyperparathyroidism

Terminology

Term	Definition
alkaline phosphatase ĂL-kă-lĭn FŎS-fă-tāz	Enzyme compound that increases in some conditions, such as parathyroidism
bilateral urolithiasis bī-LĂT-ěr-ăl ū-rō-lĭ-THĪ-ă-sĭs	Formation of kidney stones (calculi) in both kidneys
hyperlipidemia hī-pěr-lĭp-ĭ-DĒ-mē-ă	Increase in the amount of fats in the plasma
hyperparathyroidism hī-pěr-păr-ă-THĪ-roy-dĭzm	Abnormally increased activity of the parathyroids (located on both sides of the thyroid)
phosphorus FŎS-fō-rŭs	Essential mineral involved in all metabolic processes
serum calcium SĒ-rŭm KĂL-sē-ŭm	Blood test to determine the amount of calcium in the clear liquid portion of the blood

Analysis:

1. Refer to Figure 13-1. Where are the parathyroid glands located?

   There are four glands, two on each side of the thyroid gland.

2. What important function does parathyroid hormone (PTH) perform?

   Regulates calcium metabolism

3. In which way is the increase of PTH affecting this patient?

   Causing development of urinary calculi

4. What are the target organs of PTH? (Refer to Table 13-3.)

   Bones, kidneys, and small intestine

■ ■ ■ **Chapter 14–Nervous System**

Supplemental Medical Record Activity 14–1

Peripheral Neuropathy

Terminology

Term	Definition
arthralgias ăr-THRĂL-jē-ŭz	Pain in the joints
EMG	Electromyography
encephalitis ĕn-sĕf-ă-LĪ-tĭs	Inflammation of the brain
gait gāt	Style of walking
meningitis mĕn-ĭn-JĪ-tĭs	Inflammation of the meninges
otosclerosis ō-tō-sklĕ-RŌ-sĭs	Condition that is characterized by chronic, progressive deafness, especially for low tones, and caused by formation of spongy bone, especially around the oval window, with resulting ankylosis of the stapes
peripheral neuropathy pĕr-ĬF-ĕr-ăl nū-RŎP-ă-thē	Disturbance or pathological change in the peripheral nervous system
proprioception prō-prē-ō-SĔP-shŭn	Awareness of position, posture, movement, or changes in equilibrium

Analysis:

1. What are the patient's presenting complaints?

   Prolonged pain and burning in her feet, diminished proprioception, and a sense of difficulty in walking, particularly in the dark

2. Are the patient's cranial nerves intact?

   Yes, except for hearing loss

3. How was the motor system examination described?

   The patient has normal gait and station and generally good strength, coordination, and reflexes. She was able to touch her fingertips to her toes but unable to straighten up unless she bent her knees.

4. How extensive is the patient's sensory loss?

   Decreased position and vibratory sense as well as pinprick in the lower extremities, much more on the right foot up to the upper third of the shin; and just the foot and ankle on the left

Supplemental Medical Record Activity 14–2

Facial Paralysis

Terminology

Term	Definition
brainstem BRĀN-stĕm	Structure that lies deep in the center of the brain and connects with the spinal cord at the level of the medulla
cerebellar sĕr-ĕ-BĔL-ăr	Related to the cerebellum (structure that occupies the back portion of the brain and is attached to the brainstem)
dysarthric dĭs-ĂR-thrĭc	Imperfect articulation of speech
EEG	Electroencephalogram
facial paralysis FĀ-shăl pă-RĂL-ĭ-sĭs	Weakening of the facial nerve (cranial nerve VII)
MRI	Magnetic resonance imaging
nystagmus nĭs-TĂG-mŭs	Involuntary eye movement that appears jerky
uvula Ū-vū-lă	Small, fleshy mass hanging from the soft palate

Analysis:

1. Describe the patient's speech pattern.

   Speech was fluent and not disjointed.

2. What part of the patient's memory was severely impaired?

   Recent and past events

3. Why couldn't the doctor test the patient's cerebellar function?

   Because she couldn't follow two-step commands

4. How was the motor evaluation described?

   Normal muscle tone and normal strength through- out with no focal limb weakness

5. What was the diagnosis?

   Left facial paralysis which appears to be chronic, either secondary to a trauma in the past or residual for an old Bell palsy

Supplemental Medical Record Activity 14–3

Hydrocephalus

Terminology

Term	Definition
burr hole bĕr	Opening made in the skull
cephalic end sĕ-FĂL-ĭk	Pertaining to the head

Term	Definition
cm	Centimeter
craniotome KRĀ-nē-ō-tōm	Instrument to cut the bone of the skull
dura DOO-ră	Tough outer membrane covering the brain
galea GĀ-lē-ă	General term for a helmetlike structure or covering
H₂O	Chemical formula meaning water
hydrocephalus hī-drō-SĔF-ă-lŭs	Condition marked by swelling of the cerebral ventricles that is caused by obstruction in the cerebrospinal fluid pathway
ICU	Intensive care unit
lateral ventricle LĂT-ĕr-ăl VĔN-trĭ-kl	One of the cavities in the brain that is filled with cerebrospinal fluid
parietal scalp pă-RĪ-ĕ-tăl SKĂLP	Structure that forms the roof and upper part of the sides of the skull
ventriculoperitoneal shunt vĕn-trĭk-ū-lō-pĕr-ĭ-tō-NĒ-ăl SHŬNT	Surgically created passageway made of plastic tubing and one-way valves between a cerebral ventricle and the peritoneum used to drain excess cerebrospinal fluid from the brain

Analysis:

1. What instrument was used to create the burr hole?

   Craniotome

2. Where was the brain needle positioned?

   Atrium of the lateral ventricle

3. What occurred when the ventricle was entered?

   A free flow of ventricular fluid

4. What prophylactic treatment did the patient undergo?

   Systemic antibiotics and the shunt hardware soaked in bacitracin

5. What type of suture did they use to close the galea?

   2-0 Vicryl

■ ■ ■ Chapter 15–Special Senses

Supplemental Medical Record Activity 15–1

Chronic Suppurative Otitis Media

Terminology

Term	Definition
canaloplasty kă-NĂL-ō-plăs-tē	Reconstruction of the ear canal, usually to remove a bony growth
cerumen sĕ-ROO-mĕn	Waxy secretion in the ear canal

Term	Definition
eustachian tube ū-STĀ-shĕn	Tube that connects the nose and throat to the middle ear
ossicular chain ŏ-SĬK-ū-lăr	Sequence of the three ossicles
peritympanic incision pĕr-ĭ-tĭm-PĂN-ĭk ĭn-SĬ-zhŭn	Cut made around the tympanic membrane
postauricular pōst-aw-RĬK-ū-lăr	Behind the ear
purulent debris PŪR-ū-lĕnt dĕ-BRĒ	Foreign matter consisting of pus
resected rē-SĔK-tĕd	Operative procedure for the specific purpose of removal, as in shortening of the outer coat of the eye in retinal surgery
tympanic membrane perforation tĭm-PĂN-ĭk MĔM-brān pĕr-fō-RĀ-shŭn	Hole in the flat membranous structure at the end of the ear canal
tympanosclerosis tĭm-pă-nō-sklĕ-RŌ-sĭs	Hardening of the tympanic structures

Analysis:

1. Why was tympanoplasty performed?

   Because she had a perforated tympanic membrane

2. Was there an active infection?

   No, but the middle ear mucosa was mildly inflamed.

3. How did the surgeon determine if the eustachian tube was obstructed?

   By passing lacrimal probes through the opening

4. What type of incision was made?

   Peritympani

5. What type of suture did the surgeon use to close the mastoid fascia?

   3-0 Vicryl

6. Examine Figure 15-3. Notice the location of the ossicles in relation to the tympanic membrane. Which ossicle is attached to the tympanic membrane?

   Malleus

7. What item was used to support the graft in the ear canal?

   Saline-soaked Gelfoam

Supplemental Medical Record Activity 15–2

Cataract

Terminology

Term	Definition
cataract KĂT-ă-răkt	Opacities that form on the lens of the eye or the capsule that encloses the lens
BP	Blood pressure
c/d ratio	Cup to disc ratio (ophthalmology)

Term	Definition
conjunctiva kŏn-jŭnk-TĪ-vă	Thin mucous membrane that lines the inner surface of the eyelids and passes over the cornea
EOMs	Extraocular movements
exudate ĔKS-ū-dāt	Fluid or cellular debris that has deposited on tissue surfaces and is usually the result of inflammation
foveal reflexes FŌ-vē-ăl RĒ-flĕks-ĕz	Movement on the surface of a pit on the retina
gonioscopy gō-nē-ŎS-cō-pē	Examination of the angle of the posterior chamber with a gonioscope (optical instrument)
iridodonesis ĭr-ĭd-ō-dō-NĒ-sĭs	Abnormal quivering of the iris upon movement of the eye
lacrimal apparatus LĂK-rĭm-ăl ăp-ă-RĂT-ŭs	Structures making up the tear ducts
normocephalic nor-mō-sĕ-FĂL-ĭck	Pertaining to a normally shaped head
PERRLA	Pupils equal, round, and reactive to light and accommodation
retinopathy rĕt-ĭn-ŎP-ă-thē	Any disease process of the retina
sclerae SKLĔR-ē	Outermost layers of the eyeball
synechiae sĭ-NĒ-kē-ē	Adhesions at the base of the iris to the cornea
trabecular meshwork tră-BĔK-ū-lăr MĔSH-wĕrk	General term for supporting or anchoring strands of connective tissue
WD	Well-developed
WN	Well-nourished

Analysis:

1. What is causing poor vision in the left eye?

   Cataract

2. Did new glasses or pinhole improve the patient's vision?

   No, vision can no longer be improved with these two procedures.

3. When is the patient's vision the poorest?

   In bright light and under night driving conditions

4. Did the patient have any bleeding, exudates, or tears in the retinas?

   None evidenced

5. What is the diagnosis regarding glaucoma?

   Glaucoma is open angle, mild, and well controlled.

Crossword Puzzles

■ ■ ■ **Chapter 2–Suffixes**

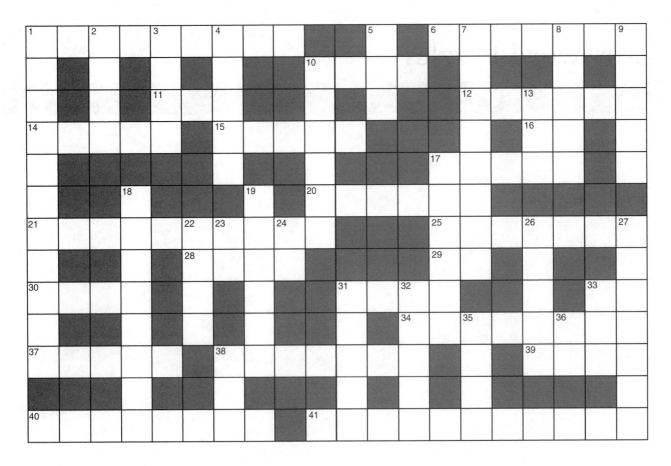

ACROSS

1. A word root plus a vowel (usually *o*) is a _____ form.
6. Add a suffix that means "relating to" to the word root *spin*.
10. Suffix that means "incision"
11. Suffix that means "specialist"
12. In "enteroscope," the combining form is _____ /_____.
14. Suffix that means "fixation (of a bone or joint)"
15. Red-breasted bird
16. Postal abbreviation for the state north of CA
17. Mother of Prince William
20. An element found at the end of a medical word
21. Add the suffix that means "study of" to the combining form *gastr/o*.
25. The student who "gets it" quickly is a fast _____.
28. A dress in New Delhi
29. You and me
30. Prayer-ending word; it means "So be it."
31. The catcher's glove
33. Postal abbreviation for Cincinnati's state

34. Add the suffix that means "tumor" to the root word *hepat*.
37. 1600 Pennsylvania Ave., the White _____
38. A gastroscope allows the physician to _____ the stomach.
39. To trade
40. The suffix -*rrhagia* means "_____ forth (of)."
41. The study of words related to anatomy, disease, and medical procedures is *medical* _____

DOWN

1. Add the suffix that means "instrument for recording" to the combining form *cardi/o*.
2. A New York baseball team
3. The suffix that means "inflammation"
4. The suffix that means "treatment" or "medicine"
5. Abbreviation for *health maintenance organization*
7. Word elements added to the beginnings of words
8. Broadway hit *The Phantom of the* _____

9. Suffix that means "instrument for examining"
10. Suffix that means "crushing"
13. Two thousand pounds
17. To weaken a solution by adding water
18. Suffix that means "narrowing, stricture"
19. Singular form of *fornices*
22. Suffix that means "abnormal condition; increase"
23. "City of Angels"
24. Abbreviation for *gastrointestinal* or nickname for a soldier
26. The foundations of medical words or the underground parts of plants
27. The suffix in *myorrhaphy* is _____.
31. Native American corn
32. The word root in *thermometer*
33. Suffix that means "tumor"
35. The suffixes -*algia* and -*dynia* mean "_____."
36. Sudden cry of pain
38. Geological term for a billion years

■ ■ ■ Chapter 3–Prefixes

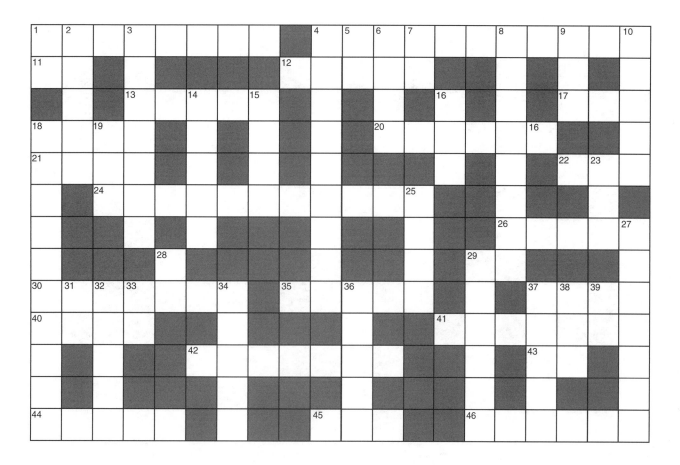

ACROSS

1. The meaning of the prefix *retro-*
4. Add a prefix to *gastrium* to form a word that means "above the stomach."
11. To form the singular of *testes*, replace the suffix *es* with _____.
12. In *extraocular,* the prefix that means "outside"
13. Prefix that means "double"
17. The suffix that means "relating to" in the word *acoustic*
18. Middle Eastern country, once ruled by the Shah
20. Prefix that means "four"
21. Sense organ used for smelling
22. In *exotoxin*, the prefix that means "outside"
24. Add the prefix that means "excessive" to *mastia*.
26. In *lithiasis*, the suffix that means "abnormal condition"
29. Abbreviation for *cubic centimeter*
30. Out of the ordinary
35. Suffix that means "act of measuring"
37. Fly high; glide

40. Prefix that means "one" or "single"
41. The suffix *-gram* means "record" or "_____."
42. Large, flightless bird
43. Abbreviation for *identification*
44. Meaning of prefix *tri-*
45. The prefix that means "together" or "joined"
46. Suffix that means "enlargement"

DOWN

1. Prefix that means "two"
2. National Leaguer from Houston
3. Organs that produce urine (combining form *nephr/o* or *ren/o*)
4. The prefix *hyper-* means "_____."
5. Abbreviation for *physical therapist*
6. Land of former dictator Saddam Hussein
7. Postal code for the Braves and Falcons
8. Add a suffix that means "pertaining to" to the root *thorac* (chest).
9. Suffix that means "specialist"
10. Prefix that means "small"

14. In *phlebotomy* ("incision of a vein"), the word root for "vein"
15. Singular form of *ova* (eggs)
16. Prefix that means "all"
18. The suffix *-scope* means "_____." for examining."
19. What is left after a fire
23. XX minus VIII
25. In *aboral*, the prefix *ab-* means "_____ from."
27. The suffix *-plasty* means "surgical repair" or "plastic _____."
28. Prefix that means "good, normal"
29. Prefix that means "around"
31. Negative
32. Both *sub-* and *infra-* mean "_____."
33. Gershwin song: *It Ain't Necessarily _____.*
34. Suffix that means "destruction"
36. Prefix that means "rapid"
37. Rock star or bee's assault
38. Suffix that means "resembling"
39. In *anesthesia*, the prefix that means "without"

■ ■ ■ Chapter 4–Body Structure

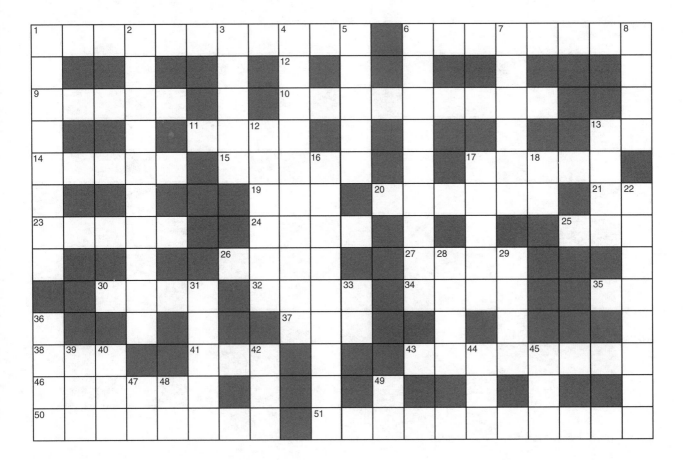

ACROSS

1. The stable internal environment of cells
6. Subjective indications of disease; what the patient feels
9. In *radiography,* the combining form that means "radiation"
10. Prediction of course and probable outcome of a disease
11. The lion's shout
13. Abbreviation for *registered nurse*
14. Bob _____ wrote *Blowin' in the Wind.*
15. Prefix that means "slow"
17. Prefix that means "same, alike"
19. Abbreviation for *magnetic resonance imaging*
20. Meaning of the prefix *peri-*
21. Type of electrical current
23. Canine, molar, or eye
24. Meaning of *-phobia*
25. A charge for professional service
26. An organ contained in the thoracic cavity
27. Earth's oldest satellite
30. Not harsh; meek
32. Alight; go ashore

34. Certain; positive
35. Abbreviation for *cardiovascular*
37. Deli item; smoked salmon
38. Little demon; mischievous child
41. Prefix that means "before, in front of"
43. Medical term that means "pertaining to the chest"
46. Opposite of *proximal*
50. The study of the cause of disease
51. Medical term that means "toward the surface of the body"

DOWN

1. Genetic inheritance
2. Medical term that means "pertaining to the area over the stomach"
3. To pulse painfully
4. Medical term that means "above the kidneys"
5. Suffix that means "forming a new opening (mouth)"
6. Recordings of ultrasonography
7. Meaning of the suffix *-toxic*
8. Objective indication of disease observed by others
12. As much as the arm can hold

13. Traveled by horseback
16. Establishment of the cause or nature of a disease
17. Mirth; what one needs a sense of
18. Postal code for Baltimore
22. Pertaining to the neck
28. Exclamation of pain
29. In *neurology,* the root that means "nerve"
31. Prefix that means "double"
33. Abbreviation for *diagnosis*
36. *Lateral* means "pertaining to the _____."
39. Cambridge, MA., home of HU and _____.
40. Abbreviation used to denote tire pressure
42. Suffix that means "pertaining to"
44. Not on
45. Circle segment
47. Familiar preposition
48. Postal code for Birmingham
49. Abbreviation for *Military Police*

■ ■ ■ Chapter 5–Integumentary System

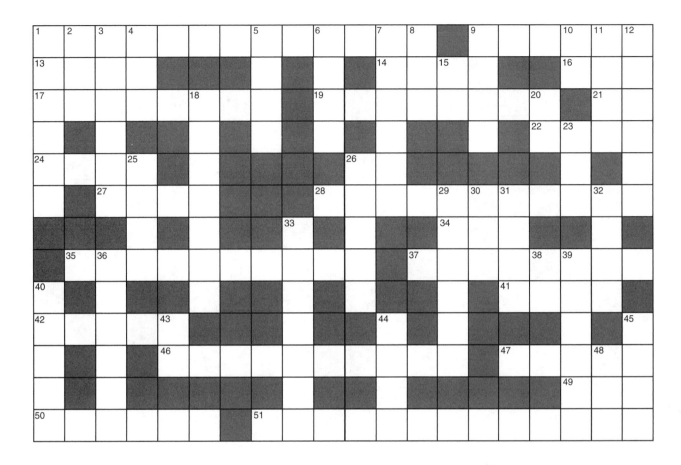

ACROSS

1. Medical term that means "softening of the nails"
9. The combining forms *mamm/o* and *mast/o* mean "_____."
13. A rhymed composition
14. Potter's raw material
16. What to do at Vail
17. *Hepatomegaly* is the medical term for an "_____ liver."
19. *Tinea pedis* is the medical term for "_____ foot."
21. Singular verb
22. Ameche, Johnson, and Corleone
24. Smallest unit of matter
26. Abbreviation for *family history*
27. A papule may be a nevus, pimple, or _____.
28. Red blood cell
34. Suffix that means "resembling"
35. Medication used to dry up secretions
37. Medical term that means "hernia containing fat"
41. Popular music; a stone
42. A lesion caused by trauma
46. Neoplasms in epithelial tissue
47. Combining form that means "gland"

49. Family member; pop's mate
50. Word root that means "chest"
51. Together, the skin, hair, nails, glands, and breasts make up the _____ system.

DOWN

1. Aida, Tosca, and Madame Butterfly
2. A common prefix that means "not"
3. Color denoted by *cirrh/o*, *jaund/o*, and *xanth/o*
4. Certified medical assistant
5. Acronym for *acquired immune deficiency syndrome*
6. The prefix *ab-* means "movement _____ from."
7. Word root that means "dry, scaly"
8. Meaning of the prefix pan
9. Unit of computer memory
10. Long-time soap opera "_____ the World Turns."
11. Meaning of the combining form *derm/o*
12. Biopsy is the excision of a small piece of _____ for microscopic examination.

15. The plural ending for some nouns ending in *a* is _____.
18. Medical term for "relating to the stomach"
20. Pierre's postal code
23. Suffix that means "relating to"
25. Word root that means "breast"
26. To foam at the mouth
29. Lifts
30. To saw wood with the grain
31. Smell
32. Converse
33. *FS* is the abbreviation for "frozen _____."
36. Combining form that means "scale"
38. Abbreviation for commanding officer
39. Inflammatory skin disease
40. *Hidr/o* is the combining form for _____.
43. Postal code for the nation's capital
44. Self-satisfied; self-righteous
45. Suffix that means "incision"
48. Abbreviation for Oslo's country

■ ■ ■ Chapter 6–Digestive System

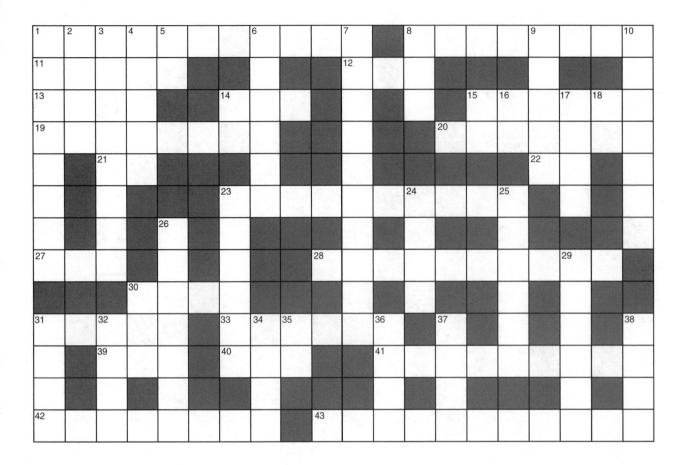

ACROSS

1. The part of the throat behind the nose
8. *Cholelithotripsy* is the medical term for "_____ a gallstone."
11. The prefix that means *outside*
12. Identity; sense of self
13. Blood coagulates to form a _____.
14. Suffix that means "tumor"
15. The suffix *-toxic* means _____.
19. To say in another way
20. Separating; ranking; classifying
21. "I told you _____."
22. Postal code for the Hawkeye state
23. Medical term that means "pain of the pylorus"
27. Prefix that means "union, together"
28. Medical term that means "relating to the epiglottis"
30. Meaning of the suffix *-dynia*
31. Term for the mass of chewed food ready to be swallowed
33. Combining form that means "tongue"
39. Suffix that means "specialist"
40. A person with *dysphagia* finds it hard to _____.
41. Medical term that means "hernia of the rectum"
42. Word root that means "bile vessel"
43. *Cholecyst/o* is the combining form for _____.

DOWN

1. Medical term that means "death of tissue"
2. Shaft on which the wheel revolves
3. Eight-sided traffic symbol
4. Combing form that means "straight"
5. Abbreviation for *posteroanterior*
6. Cure or treatment
7. Recordings of x-ray images on Xerox paper
8. Word root that means "colon"
9. Caribbean nation, capital Port au Prince
10. Combining form that means "gum"
14. Latin word for "mouth" or "opening"
15. Abbreviation for *postoperative*
16. Word root that means "mouth"
17. Word root that means "saliva" or "salivary gland"
18. Not off
23. Dive or dip suddenly
24. Suffix that means "the study of"
25. Combining form that means "anterior, front"
26. Medical term that means "lack of breast"
29. Word root that means "appendix"
30. The combining form *py/o* means "_____."
31. Word root that means "cheek"
32. Combining form that means "fat"
34. Word root that means "lip"
35. Abbreviation for *occupational therapist*
36. The medical term that means "pertaining to the mouth"
37. Crust over a sore or wound
38. Meaning of the suffix *-phobia*

■ ■ ■ Chapter 7–Respiratory System

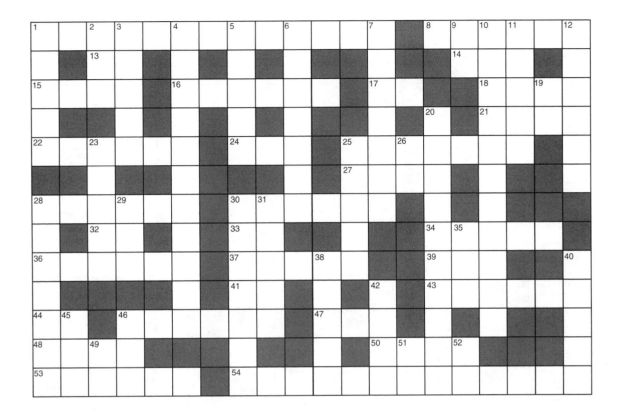

ACROSS

1. Sudden contractions of the bronchial passages
8. The voice box
13. Postal abbreviation for Iowa
14. Astrological lion
15. Abbreviation for *acute respiratory distress syndrome*
16. "The _____ and the Pauper"
17. Abbreviation for *respiratory disease*
18. The combining form *derm/o* means "_____."
21. Nuisance; annoying one
22. Classic Disney dog movie "Old _____."
24. Tenth month, in short
25. Resembling a gland
27. Suffix that means "instrument to cut"
28. Term that means "absence of oxygen in the tissues"
30. Reply
32. Abbreviation for *myocardial infarction*
33. Abbreviation for *not applicable*
34. Night-flying insects
36. The act of seeing
37. Combining form that means "straight"
39. Combining form that means "oxygen"
41. Compass direction
43. Medical term that means "upper respiratory infection"
44. Latin for *mouth*
46. Amulets; lucky pieces
47. Abbreviation for *upper respiratory infection*
48. Combining form that means "lobe"
50. Word root that means "calcium"
53. *Hypoxemia* is "deficiency of _____ in the blood."
54. Medical term that means "excision of an adrenal gland"

DOWN

1. Prefix that means "slow"
2. Suffix that means "resembling"
3. Medical term that means "pertaining to the nose"
4. Excessive CO_2 in the blood
5. Combining form that means "breathe"
6. Medical term that means "accumulation of fluid in the peritoneal cavity"
7. Abnormal breath sound due to obstruction of air passages
9. Adjective suffix that means "pertaining to"
10. The lungs are the major organs of the _____ system.
11. Joined together, like oxen
12. Combining form that means "yellow"
19. Abbreviation for *intercostal space*
20. Medical term that means "hernia of the lung"
23. Machines for weaving
25. Combining form that means "incomplete" or "imperfect"
26. Dorothy's Auntie _____
28. Combining form that means "alveolus"
29. XXIV divided by II
30. Medical term that means "loss of the sense of smell"
31. Medical term that means "nostrils"
35. Combining form that means "oxygen"
38. United States Senate and _____ of Representatives.
40. Prefix that means "fast"
42. Transparent mineral
45. Before the Yankees, the Babe played for the Red _____.
46. A tooth on the rim of a gear
49. Preposition that means "near"
51. Postal code for Mobile
52. Metric abbreviation; approximately 1 mL

■ ■ ■ Chapter 8–Cardiovascular System

ACROSS

1. The heart and blood vessels make up the _____ system.
8. Award in the form of a metallic disk
11. Combining form that means "anus"
12. Fleets
15. Combining form that means "back (of body), behind, posterior"
16. Abbreviation for *electrocardiograph*
18. Abbreviation for *aortic stenosis*
19. Homonym for "a needle pulling thread"
20. Abbreviation for *gastrointestinal*
21. Apprehend; nab
22. Strapped; or smacked
23. Throb felt in the arterial wall
26. Word root that means "ileum"
27. Word root that means "clot"
28. Strike with open hand
31. First rib donor; Eve's mate
33. Combining form that means "blood"
34. Sac containing the heart
40. State of the Phillies and the Pirates
41. Word root that means "yellow"
42. Abbreviation for *very low-density lipoprotein*

44. Open, unobstructed
46. Fish or word root that means "wrist"
48. Combining form that means "atrium"
49. Surgical removal of the innermost layer of the artery

DOWN

1. The right atrium is a _____ of the heart.
2. Relaxation phase of the heartbeat
3. Combining form that means "blood vessel"
4. The smallest blood vessel
5. Nevada city: _____ Vegas
6. Prefix that means "against"
7. Fish eggs
8. Medical term that means "pertaining to the muscles of the heart"
9. To eat and drink sparingly, perhaps to lower blood cholesterol levels
10. Not heavy
13. Prefix that means "bad"
14. Abbreviation for *atrial septal defect*

17. Cardiac catheterization, for short
20. Leaders, advisors
24. Adjective for a valve in the pulmonary artery that literally means "resembling a half moon"
25. Harsh and rigid or the rear of a boat
28. A passage between two blood vessels or between two sides of the heart
29. Prefix that means "on both sides"
30. Author of "The Raven": Edgar Allan _____
31. Temporary stopping of breath
32. Suffix that means "suture"
35. Abbreviation for *cardiovascular*
36. Org. for recovering alcoholics
37. Godlike
38. Combining form that means "black"
39. Prefix that means "outside"
43. Postal code for the White House
44. Prefix that means "before"
45. Jack's youngest brother, Senator Kennedy
47. Abbreviation for *myocardial infarction*

■ ■ ■ Chapter 9–Blood, Lymph, and Immune Systems

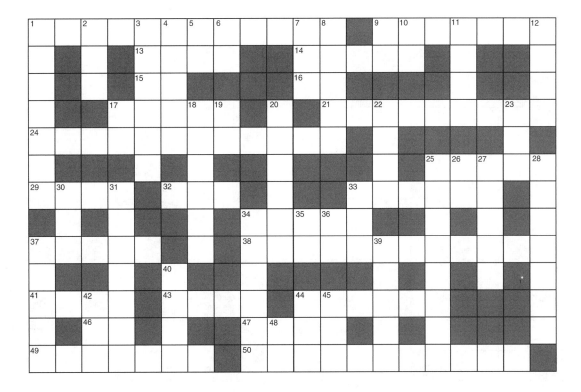

ACROSS

1. Smallest formed elements in the blood; platelets
9. Combining form that means "granule"
13. Abbreviation for *eyes, ears, nose, and throat*
14. Word root that means "sternum"
15. Cellist YoYo _____
16. Providence postal code
17. Word root that means "shape"
21. Medical term that means "tumors of the lymphatic system"
24. Another term that means tissue fluid: "_____ fluid"
25. Sharing expenses is known as "going _____ treat"
29. Detergent
32. Prefix that means "same or equal"
33. Combining form that means "dawn (rose-colored)"
34. Plasma minus fibrinogen is known as "blood _____"
37. Suffix that means "separation, destruction, loosening"
38. Blood and lymph are essential for _____ gases, nutrients, and waste to and from body cells
41. Prefix that means "middle"
43. Combining form that means "fungus"
44. Opposite of *reject*

46. Postal code for the Windy City
47. Combining form that means "nucleus"
49. B-cells are responsible for _____ immunity
50. Red blood cell

DOWN

1. Lymphatic tissue in the mouth and throat
2. Abbreviation for *erythrocyte*
3. Some activated T cells and B cells act as _____ cells in specific immunity.
4. The NFL's Chicago _____
5. Not off
6. Abbreviation for *computerized tomography*
7. Abbreviation for *erythrocyte sedimentation rate*
8. The suffix *-stasis* means "standing _____."
9. Abbreviation for *grain*
10. Abbreviation for *registered nurse*
11. Combining form that means *nose*
12. Suffix that means *condition of*
17. He/him, she/her, I/_____
18. Suffix that means "prolapse, downward displacement"
19. Honolulu postal code
20. Disagree

22. Combining form that means "one"
23. Section of a circle
25. Agent that increases the secretion of urine
26. International peacekeeping org.
27. Suffix that means "poison"
28. Malignant disease of the lymph nodes, spleen, and liver: "_____ disease"
30. Suffix that means "pertaining to"
31. Combining form that means "varied, irregular"
33. Abbreviation for *emergency medical service*
34. Common synonym for *cerebrovascular accident*
35. Abbreviation for *right atrium*
36. Abbreviation for *ulnar nerve*
37. Interstitial fluid in blind-ended capillaries
39. Word root that means "pleura"
40. Suffix that means "blood"
42. Not bright
44. Suffix that means "pertaining to"
45. Word root that means "cell"
48. Little Rock postal code

■ ■ ■ Chapter 10–Musculoskeletal System

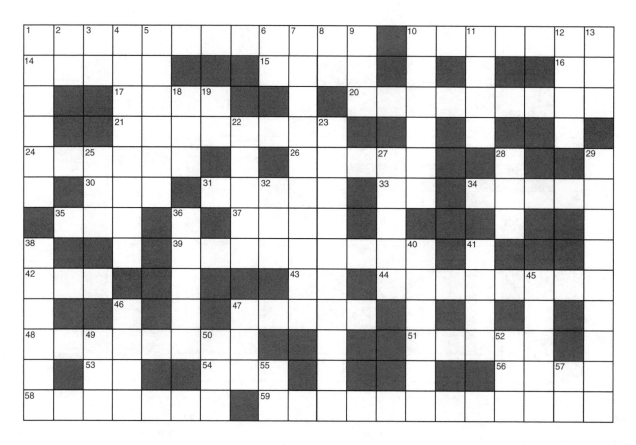

ACROSS

1. Relating to paralysis of all four extremities
10. Combining form that means "condyle"
14. The meaning of the prefix *sub-*
15. Roentgenogram
16. Abbreviation for *active resistance*
17. Sondheim musical: *Little _____ of Horrors*
20. Excision of a tendon
21. Combining form that means "heel bone"
24. Surface; come out
26. Abbreviation for *nonsteroidal anti-inflammatory drug*
30. Illusion: "_____ in the sky"
31. Banquet; great meal
33. Org. for recovering alcoholics
34. Combining form that means "spinal cord"
35. *Cost/o* is the combining form that means "_____."
37. Light beer: "Bud _____"
39. Lateral curvature of the spine
42. Abbreviation for *hematocrit*
43. Trucker's radio, abbrev.
44. Suffix that means "narrowing, stricture"

47. The most distal joint of the lower extremity
48. Movement of a bone around its longitudinal axis
51. Old term for *redness due to inflammation*
53. Madison postal code
54. The combining form *rhabd/o* means "_____ shaped (striated)."
56. Word root that means "breast"
58. Combining form that means "cartilage"
59. Radiographic examination of a joint

DOWN

1. To shake or tremble
2. International peacekeeping org.
3. The era following B.C.
4. Portray in words
5. Suffix that means "bursting forth (of)"
6. Prefix that means "out" or "out from"
7. Type of fracture, common in children, in which the bone is partially bent and partially broken
8. Postal code for Iowa
9. Word root for "cell"
10. The Maple Leaf nation
11. Meaning of the combining form *cervic/o*

12. What Lady Liberty holds beside her golden door
13. Suffix that means "pertaining to"
18. Suffix that means "small, minute"
19. Abbreviation for *personal computer*
22. Combining form that means "incomplete; imperfect"
23. Bone-forming cell
25. Prefix that means "above, upon"
27. Suffix that means "abnormal condition (produced by something specified)"
28. Combining form that means "muscle"
29. Term for surgically creating a new opening in the colon
32. To be ill
36. Word root that means "ischium"
38. Word root that means "chest"
40. Combining form that means "breast-bone"
41. One who looks down on others
45. To secure with a belt or band
46. Meaning of the suffix *-dynia*
47. Combining form that means "anus"
49. Meaning of the prefix *bi-*
50. Combining form that means "mouth"
52. Suffix that means "tumor"
55. Abbreviation for *district attorney*
57. Abbreviation for *marital history*

■ ■ ■ Chapter 11–Genitourinary System

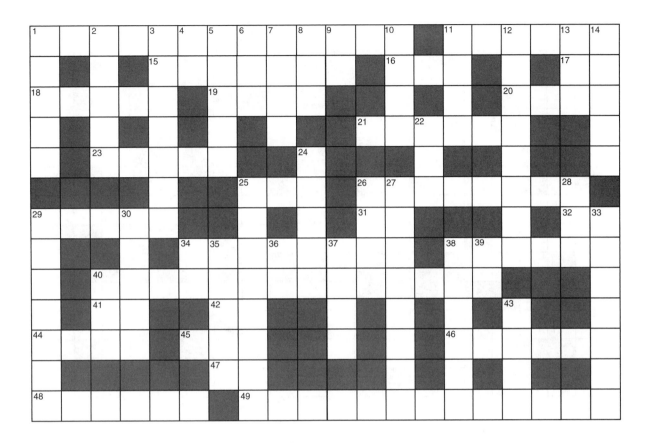

ACROSS

1. Cowper's glands are also known as "_____ glands."
11. Combining form that means "kidney"
15. Suffix that means "bursting forth (of)"
16. Suffix that means "small"
17. Abbreviation for *ultraviolet*
18. Relating to the eye or to sight
19. Suffix that means "inflammation"
20. Word root that means "bone"
21. Furniture or committee heads
23. Combining form that means "scanty"
25. Abbreviation for *benign prostatic hypertrophy*
26. Determine worth
29. Combining form that means "sugar, sweetness"
31. Bangor postal code
32. Prefix that means "good"
34. Medical term for "bed-wetting"
38. More relaxed
40. Inflammation of the renal pelvis and kidney tissue
41. Abbreviation for *retrograde pyelogram*

42. Successor to LP
44. Robert Burns was one
45. Abbreviation for *urinary tract infection*
46. Suffix that means "formation, growth"
47. Not off
48. The suffix *-rrhaphy* means "_____."
49. Pertaining to the genitals and urinary system

DOWN

1. Meaning of the combining form *hem/o*
2. Combining form that means "stone"
3. Combining form that means "testes"
4. Word root that means "urine"
5. Combining form that means "nose"
6. Meaning of the combining form *phag/o*
7. Acronym for the beginning of the weekend
8. Not hers
9. Abbreviation for *right atrium*
10. Nessie, the _____ Ness monster
11. Plural of *nevus*

12. Combining form that means "prostate gland"
13. Deep groove
14. Kilns
22. Movie star Gardner
24. Source of the wolf's disguise
25. Leaping
26. Arab ruler
27. Combining form that means "seminal vesicle"
28. Bigfoot's shoe width
29. Suffix that means "origin"
30. Word root that means "hidden"
33. Pertaining to urine
34. Elevated train, for short
35. Combining form that means "night"
36. Abbreviation for *regarding*
37. "_____ 'til you drop."
38. Not as stiff
39. Per Joint Commission, abbreviation that is no longer acceptable for *left eye*
40. Prefix that means "before, in front of"
43. Meaning of the suffix *-dynia*

■ ■ ■ Chapter 12–Female Reproductive System

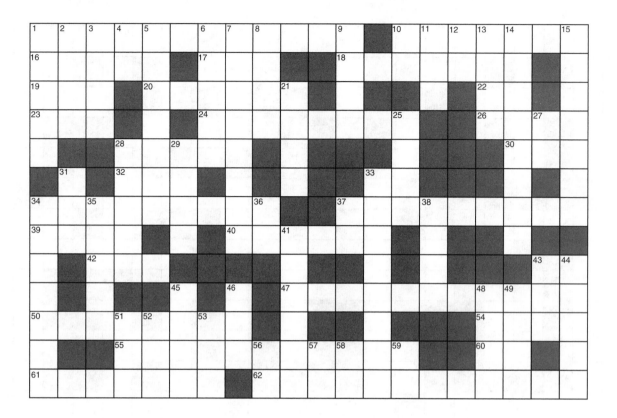

ACROSS

1. The uterus is a major organ of the female _____ system.
10. Word root that means "fallopian tube"
16. Combining form that means "gland"
17. Prefix that means "new"
18. Composed of soil
19. Bear's abode
20. Meaning of combining form *toxic/o*
22. Spielberg alien
23. Abbreviation for *Immigration and Naturalization Service*
24. Gifted
26. Word root that means "pelvis"
28. Model; one who sits for an artist
30. Baseball stat
32. Combining form that means "urine'
33. Abbreviation for *bowel movement*
34. Oviducts are also known as "_____ tubes."
37. Medical term that means "woman who has borne one child"
39. Suffix that means "inflammation"
40. Combining form that means "kidney"
42. Word root that means "middle"
43. Postal code for Bangor
47. Medical term that means "loosening of the nail bed"
50. A specialist in optical equipment

54. Grain for horses
55. Vaginal fungal infection
60. Abbreviation for *kilogram*
61. Painful urination
62. Medical term that means "porous bones"

DOWN

1. Combining form that means "radiation"
2. Adam and Eve's first address
3. Writing devices
4. Abbreviation for *registered nurse*
5. Combining form that means "ovary"
6. Merge, wed, come together
7. Surgery to deliver a baby: "_____ section."
8. Utensil, implement
9. Abbreviation for *eyes, ears, nose, throat*
10. Spanish equivalent of "Mr."
11. Abbreviation for *acute tubular necrosis*
12. Abbreviation for *luteinizing hormone*
13. Chick's first cry
14. Opposite of *external*
15. Medical term that means "pregnant woman"
21. The cervix is the "_____" of the uterus.

25. Actress Moore
27. Abbreviation for *pound*
28. Rhythmic throb felt in artery
29. What the frosh becomes
31. Meaning of combining form *lip/o*
33. Combining form that means "bronchus"
34. Resembling fiber
35. Boundary
36. Omaha postal code
37. Abbreviation for *pregnancy rate*
38. Combining form that means "menses"
41. Suffix that means "falling, dropping"
43. Big school in Cambridge; not HU
44. Ems, kews, teas, and _____ .
45. Revealing skirt
46. Prefix that means "one"
48. John's widow, Sean's mother
49. Droops
51. Abbreviation for *intensive care unit*
52. Four-wheeled vehicle
53. Abbreviation for *Americans with Disabilities Act*
56. "Just _____ It."
57. Abbreviation for *athletic trainer*
58. Oregon to Florida direction
59. Abbreviation for *specific gravity:* "_____ gr"

■ ■ ■ Chapter 13–Endocrine System

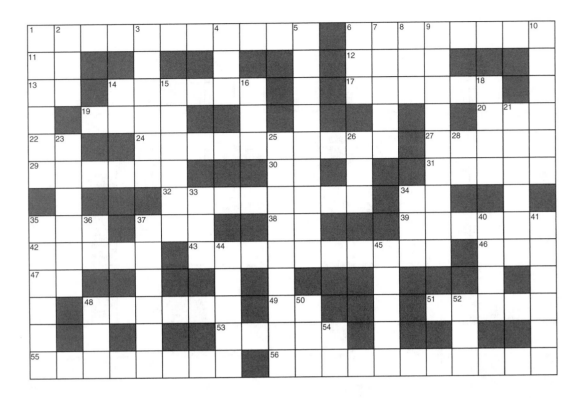

ACROSS

1. Hormone from the adrenal cortex
6. Meaning of suffix -cele
11. Abbreviation for *diabetes insipidus*
12. Nautical greeting
13. Abbreviation for *retrograde pyelogram*
14. Word root that means "skin"
17. Less bright
19. Biblical boat builder
20. Legal assoc.
22. Postal code for Raleigh
24. Instrument for viewing bacteria and cells
27. Wished, desired
29. Word root that means "ovary"
30. Abbreviation for *operating room*
31. Combining form that means "straight"
32. Computerized tomography is a method of _____ body planes with x-rays.
34. Abbreviation for giant American carmaker
35. Combining form that means "ear"
37. Beach Boys song: "My Little _____"
38. Fonda movie: _____ *Golden Pond*
39. Meaning of the suffix -*phagia*
42. Nickname for a southpaw

43. Specialized pancreatic cells: "the islets of _____"
46. Abbreviation for *low-density lipoprotein*
47. Abbreviation for *diagnosis*
48. In chess, made the first move
49. Abbreviation for *analytical reagent*
51. *Inguinal*: "pertaining to the _____"
53. Meaning of the prefix *tachy*-
55. Combining form that means "thyroid gland"
56. The state of equilibrium in the body's internal environment

DOWN

1. Combining form that means "adrenal glands"
2. Meaning of the combining form *labi/o*
3. Combining form that means "scale"
4. Word root that means "kidney"
5. The _____ system works with the nervous system to maintain homeostasis.
6. Blue, down in the dumps
7. Meaning of the combining form *leuk/o*
8. Abbreviation for *extraocular movement*

9. Neoplasms of the lymphatic system
10. Combining form that means "sex glands"
14. Denver postal code
15. Meaning of the suffix -*dipsia*
16. Prefix that means "outside"
18. Engrossed
21. Meaning of *poster/o*
23. Each adrenal gland consists of an outer _____ and inner medulla.
25. Medical term that means "instrument used to record sound waves"
26. Bacon on the hoof
28. Word root that means "mouth"
33. Word root that means "colon"
34. Suffix that means "to produce"
35. Most aged
36. Possessive preposition
37. Combining form that means "woman"
40. Combining form that means "ileum"
41. The endocrine _____ release secretions directly into the bloodstream.
44. Combining form that means "male"
45. Combining form that means "gland"
48. Suffix that means "pertaining to"
50. Brazil's largest city, for short
52. Abbreviation for *ribonucleic acid*
54. Diabetes mellitus, for short

■ ■ ■ Chapter 14–Nervous System

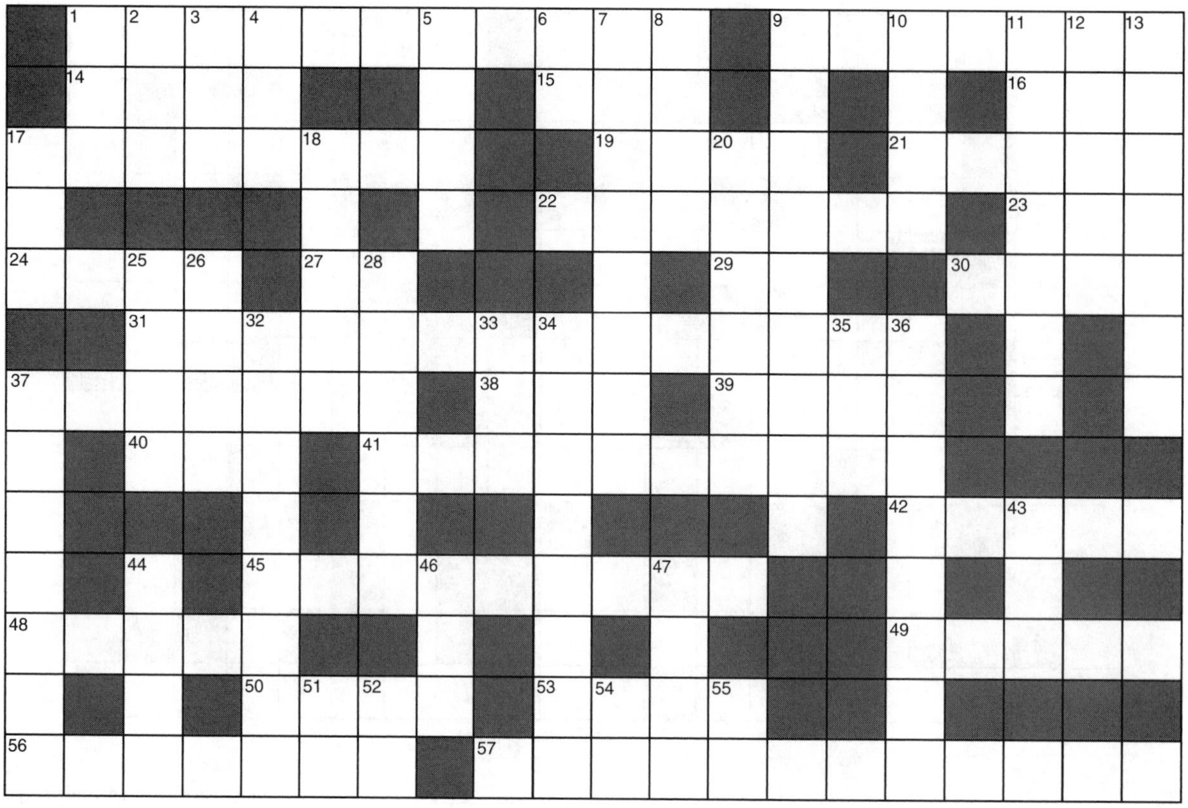

[Crossword puzzle grid]

ACROSS

1. Irregular brain wave tracings
9. Suffix that means "movement"
14. Cat quote
15. Pro football org.
16. Kind of dance
17. *Narc/o* is the combining form that means "_____."
19. Meaning of the prefix *quadri-*
21. To splash with liquid
22. Puts the packaging back together
23. Woody's ex
24. Combining form that means "extremity"
27. Abbreviation for *Nova Scotia*
29. "_____, phone home."
30. Bulk, magnitude, size
31. Drugs used to control brain seizures
37. Room to avoid for the heat-sensitive
38. Word root that means "kidney"
39. Volcano in Sicily
40. Mediterranean or Caspian
41. *Lithotripsy* is _____ of stones or calculi
42. Prefix that means "between"
45. Home of the dingo, platypus, and kangaroo
48. Elite; what rises to the top of the milk
49. Prefix that means "rapid"
50. Cosmetically challenged; very unattractive
53. Combining form that means "glue"
56. Suffix that means "partial paralysis"
57. Structure immediately below the thalamus

DOWN

1. Abbreviation for *atomic mass unit*
2. Abbreviation for *rapid eye movement*
3. Steal
4. Abbreviation for someone from Hawaii
5. Master of ceremonies; emcee
6. Hoosier postal code
7. _____ nerves conduct signals toward the central nervous system.
8. Meaning of the prefix *brady-*
9. Corneal infection
10. "Untouchable"; he got Capone
11. Meaning of combining form *gastr/o*
12. Suffix that means "abnormal condition (produced by something specified)"
13. Inability to speak
17. Abbrev. for *National Institute on Aging*
18. Bert's pal; friend of Big Bird
20. Meaning of the combining form *ureter/o*
25. First ones off the sinking ship
26. At one time; formerly
28. Taste, touch, hearing, sight, and sound
32. Interbrain structure that processes sensory stimuli (except for smell)
33. Abbreviation for *Irish Republican Army*
34. Sluggishness or slow response
35. Cable News Network
36. A plane of the body
37. Meaning of the combining form *patell/o*
43. Spasmodic muscular contraction
44. Word root that means "nerve"
46. Fatal congenital enzyme deficiency:" _____-Sachs disease"
47. Combining form that means "ilium"
51. Abbreviation for *gastrointestinal*
52. Short for "left side"
54. Abbreviation for *lumbar puncture*
55. Abbreviation for *occupational therapist*

■ ■ ■ Chapter 15–Special Senses

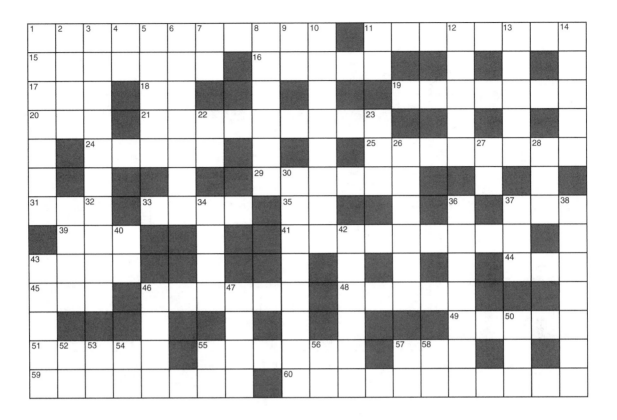

ACROSS

1. Medical term that means "excessive turning"
11. Combining form that means "eyelid"
15. *Myring/o* is the combining form for "_____."
16. Hitch digit
17. Plural of *am*
18. 60 min = 1 _____
19. Light-sensitive inner layers of eyes
20. Abbreviation for *registered nurses*
21. Catching or tangling up in a net
24. The optic nerve carries impulses to the _____.
25. Suffix that means "feeling"
29. Leiomyomas are tumors of _____ muscle tissue.
31. Initials for muscle car?
33. Homely, unattractive
35. Abbreviation for *emergency room*
37. "Extraocular movement," for short
39. Prefix that means "above, upon"
41. Involuntary, jerky eye movement
43. Suffix that means "abnormal condition of"
44. Prefix that means "before, in front of"
45. School group (abbrev.)
46. Charles, _____ of Wales

48. Suffix that means "abnormal condition" or "presence of"
49. Word root that means "ischium"
51. Combining form that means "iris"
55. Outer layer of the eye
57. Suffix that means "to produce"
59. Opaque formation on the lens of the eye
60. Inflammation of the fallopian tube (or eustachian tube)

DOWN

1. Presbyacusis: "_____ loss"
2. Strand of fiber
3. Age-related nearsightedness
4. Short for Edward
5. Suffix that means "flow"
6. Meaning of the suffix *-tropia*
7. Classified ad abbreviation for *room*
8. Suffix that means "prolapse, downward displacement"
9. Abbreviation for *infectious hepatitis*
10. Otoscopy: visual examination of the external _____ canal
11. Pellet for air rifle
12. Eyewear for Long John Silver
13. Mother's sisters
14. Suffix that means "vision"
22. Postal code for the Twin Cities

23. Acquire
26. Clips the wool of a sheep
27. Prefix that means "good"
28. Prefix that means "equal"
30. _____ disease: progressive disorder of the labyrinth, marked by vertigo and tinnitus (possessive form)
32. Exam, quiz
34. Word root that means "lip"
36. Entertaining, witty
37. Sixth sense
38. Drugs that cause constriction of the pupils
40. Third-person singular of 17 Across
42. *Myel/o* is the combining form for "_____ cord."
43. Pertaining to the eye or vision
46. Meaning of the prefix *mal-*
47. Word root that means "night"
50. Word root that means "cell"
52. Abbreviation for *right atrium*
53. Tina Turner tune: "What's Love Got to Do with _____?"
54. Abbreviation for *developmental age*
55. Postal code for Charleston
56. Abbreviation for *rheumatoid arthritis*
57. Short for *gastrointestinal*
58. Ell, em, _____, owe, pea

CHAPTER 2–SUFFIXES

■ Answer Key

C	O	M	B	I	N	I	N	G			H		S	P	I	N	O	U	S
A		E		A		T	O	M	Y		R			P			C
R		T		I	S	T		R	O			E	N	T	E	R	O
D	E	S	I	S		R	O	B	I	N			F		O	R		P
I				Y			P			D	I	A	N	A		E
O			S			F		S	U	F	F	I	X			
G	A	S	T	R	O	L	O	G	Y			L	E	A	R	N	E	R
R			E		S	A	R	I			U	S		O		R
A	M	E	N		I		N		M	I	T	T			O		O	H
P			O		S		I			A	H	E	P	A	T	O	M	A
H	O	U	S	E		E	X	A	M	I	N	E		A		S	W	A	P
			I			O			Z		R		I			H
B	U	R	S	T	I	N	G		T	E	R	M	I	N	O	L	O	G	Y

CHAPTER 3–PREFIXES

■ Answer Key

1 B	2 A	C	3 K	W	A	R	D	■	4 E	5 P	6 I	7 G	A	S	8 T	R	9 I	U	10 M
11 I	S	■	I	■	■	■	■	12 E	X	T	R	A	■	■	H	■	S	■	I
■	T	■	13 D	I	14 P	L	15 O	■	C	■	A	■	16 P	■	O	■	17 T	I	C
18 I	R	19 A	N	■	H	■	V	■	E	■	20 Q	U	A	D	R	16 I	■	■	R
21 N	O	S	E	■	L	■	U	■	S	■	■	■	N	■	A	■	22 E	23 X	O
S	■	24 H	Y	P	E	R	M	A	S	T	I	25 A	■	■	C	■	■	I	■
T	■	■	S	■	B	■	■	■	I	■	■	W	■	■	26 I	A	S	I	27 S
R	■	■	■	28 E	■	■	■	■	V	■	■	A	■	29 C	C	■	■	■	U
30 U	31 N	32 U	33 S	U	A	34 L	■	35 M	E	36 T	R	Y	■	I	■	37 S	38 O	39 A	R
40 M	O	N	O	■	■	Y	■	■	■	A	■	■	41 W	R	I	T	I	N	G
E	■	D	■	■	42 O	S	T	R	I	C	H	■	■	C	■	43 I	D	■	E
N	■	E	■	■	■	I	■	■	■	H	■	■	■	U	■	N	■	■	R
44 T	H	R	E	E	■	S	■	■	45 S	Y	N	■	■	46 M	E	G	A	L	Y

CHAPTER 4–BODY STRUCTURE

■ Answer Key

1			2			3		4		5			6		7				8
H	O	M	E	O	S	T	A	S	I	S		S	Y	M	P	T	O	M	S
E			P			H		12 U		T		O			O				I
9 R	A	D	I	O		R		10 P	R	O	G	N	O	S	I	S		13	G
E			G		11 R	O	12 A	R		M		O			S			R	N
14 D	Y	L	A	N		15 B	R	A	16 D	Y		G		17 H	O	18 M	E	O	
I			S				19 M	R	I		20 A	R	O	U	N	D		21 D	22 C
23 T	O	O	T	H		24 F	E	A	R		A		M			25 F	E	E	E
Y			R		26 L	U	N	G		27 M	O	28 O	29 N					35	R
		30 M	I	L	D		31	32 L	A	N	33 D	34 S	U	R	E			C	V
36 S			C		I			37 L	O	X			C		U				I
38 I	39 M	40 P			41 P	R	42 O		S			43 T	H	O	44 R	A	45 C	I	C
46 D	I	S	47 T	48 A	L		R		I		49 M			F		R			A
50 E	T	I	O	L	O	G	Y		51 S	U	P	E	R	F	I	C	I	A	L

CHAPTER 5–INTEGUMENTARY SYSTEM

■ Answer Key

¹O	²N	³Y	⁴C	H	O	M	⁵A	L	⁶A	C	⁷I	⁸A		⁹B	R	E	A	¹⁰S	¹¹T	¹²T
¹³P	O	E	M				I		W		¹⁴C	L	A	Y			¹⁶S	K	I
¹⁷E	N	L	A	¹⁸R	G	E	D		¹⁹A	T	H	L	E	T	E	²⁰S		²¹I	S
R		L		A		S		Y		T			E		²²D	O	²³N	S
²⁴A	T	O	²⁵M	S					²⁶F	H					R		U
S		²⁷W	A	R	T			²⁸E	R	Y	T	²⁹H	³⁰R	³¹O	C	Y	³²T	E
			S	R			³³S		O			³⁴O	I	D			A
	³⁵A	³⁶S	T	R	I	N	G	E	N	T		³⁷L	I	P	O	C	³⁸E	³⁹L	E
⁴⁰S		Q		C			C		H			S		⁴¹R	O	C	K
⁴²W	O	U	N	⁴³D			T			⁴⁴S		T			Z		⁴⁵T
E		A		⁴⁶C	A	R	C	I	N	O	M	A	S		⁴⁷A	D	E	⁴⁸N	O
A		M					O			U						⁴⁹M	O	M
⁵⁰T	H	O	R	A	C		⁵¹I	N	T	E	G	U	M	E	N	T	A	R	Y

CHAPTER 6–DIGESTIVE SYSTEM

■ Answer Key

¹N	²A	³S	⁴O	⁵P	H	A	⁶R	Y	N	⁷X		⁸C	R	U	S	⁹H	I	N	¹⁰G
¹¹E	X	T	R	A			E			¹²E	G	O			A				I
¹³C	L	O	T			¹⁴O	M	A		R		L		¹⁵P	¹⁶O	I	¹⁷S	¹⁸O	N
¹⁹R	E	P	H	R	A	S	E			O			²⁰S	O	R	T	I	N	G
O		²¹S	O			D			G			²²I	A					I
S		I		²³P	Y	L	O	R	A	²⁴L	G	I	A				V
I		G		²⁶A		L			A	O		N				O
²⁷S	Y	N		M		U		²⁸E	P	I	G	L	O	T	T	²⁹A	L
			³⁰P	A	I	N			H		Y			E		P
³¹B	O	³²L	U	S			³³G	³⁴L	O	³⁵S	O	³⁶S		³⁷S		R	P	³⁸F
U		³⁹I	S	T		⁴⁰E	A	T			⁴¹R	E	C	T	O	C	E	L	E
C		P	I			B			A		A			N	A
⁴²C	L	O	L	A	N	G	I		⁴³G	A	L	L	B	L	A	D	D	E	R

CHAPTER 7–RESPIRATORY SYSTEM

■ Answer Key

¹B	R	²O	³N	C	⁴H	O	⁵S	P	A	⁶S	M	⁷S		⁸L	⁹A	R	¹⁰Y	¹¹N	¹²X
R		¹³I	A	Y		P		S		T				¹⁴L	E	O			A
¹⁵A	R	D	S		¹⁶P	R	I	N	C	E		¹⁷R	D			¹⁸S	K	¹⁹I	N
D		A		E	R		I			I			²⁰P		²¹P	E	S	T	H
²²Y	E	²³L	L	E	R		²⁴O	C	T		²⁵A	D	²⁶E	N	O	I	D		O
		O		C				E		²⁷T	O	M	E	R					O
²⁸A	N	O	²⁹X	I	A		³⁰A	³¹N	S	W	E	R		U			A		
L		³²M	I		P		³³N	A			L			³⁴M	³⁵O	T	H	S	
³⁶V	I	S	I	O	N		³⁷O	R	T	³⁸H	O		³⁹O	X	O				⁴⁰T
E				I		⁴¹S	E		O		⁴²M		⁴³C	O	R	Y	Z	A	
⁴⁴O	⁴⁵S		⁴⁶C	H	A	R	M	S		⁴⁷U	R	I		E		Y			C
⁴⁸L	O	⁴⁹B	O			I			S		⁵⁰C	⁵¹A	L	⁵²C					H
⁵³O	X	Y	G	E	N		⁵⁴A	D	R	E	N	A	L	E	C	T	O	M	Y

CHAPTER 8–CARDIOVASCULAR SYSTEM

■ Answer Key

1 C	A	R	2 D	I	O	3 V	A	S	4 C	U	5 L	6 A	7 R		8 M	E	9 D	A	10 L
H			I			A			A		11 A	N	O		T		I		I
12 A	R	13 M	A	D	14 A	S			15 P	O	S	T	E	R	O		16 E	17 C	G
M		18 A	S		19 S	O		20 G	I			I			21 C	A	T	C	H
22 B	E	L	T	E	D		23 P	U	L	24 S	E		25 S		A				T
E			O					26 I	L	E			27 T	H	R	O	M	B	
R		28 S	L	29 A	30 P		31 A	D	A	M			E		D				32 R
		33 H	E	M	O		34 P	E	R	I	35 C	36 A	R	37 D	I	U	38 M		R
39 E		U		40 P	E	N	N	S	Y	L	V	A	N	I	A		E		H
41 X	A	N	T	H			E			U				42 V	L	43 D	L		A
T		T		I		44 P	A	45 T	E	N	T			I		46 C	A	R	P
R			47 M			R		E		A				N			N		H
48 A	T	R	I	O		49 E	N	D	A	R	T	E	R	E	C	T	O	M	Y

CHAPTER 9—BLOOD, LYMPH, AND IMMUNE SYSTEMS
■ **Answer Key**

¹T	²H	R	³O	⁴M	⁵B	⁶O	C	Y	⁷T	⁸E	S		⁹G	¹⁰R	A	N	¹¹U	L	¹²O
O	B		¹³E	E	N	T			¹⁴S	T	E	R	N		A			S
N		C		¹⁵M	A			¹⁶R	I					A			¹²³ S	I
S			¹⁷M	O	R	¹⁸P	¹⁹H		²⁰D		²¹L	²²Y	M	P	H	O	M	²³A	S
²⁴I	N	T	E	R	S	T	I	T	I	A	L		O					R
L			Y		O			F				N		²⁵D	²⁶U	²⁷T	C	²⁸H
²⁹S	³⁰O	A	³¹P		³²I	S	O		F		³³E	O	S	I	N	O		O
	R		O		I		³⁴S	E	³⁵R	³⁶U	M		U		X		D
³⁷L	Y	S	I	S		S		³⁸T	R	A	N	S	³⁹P	O	R	T	I	N	G
Y		K		⁴⁰E			R					L		E		C		K
⁴¹M	E	⁴²D	I		⁴³M	Y	C	O		⁴⁴A	⁴⁵C	C	E	P	T		I
P		⁴⁶I	L	I		⁴⁷K	⁴⁸A	R	Y		U		I			N
⁴⁹H	U	M	O	R	A	L		⁵⁰E	R	Y	T	H	R	O	C	Y	T	E

CHAPTER 10–MUSCULOSKELETAL SYSTEM

■ Answer Key

Q	U	A	D	R	I	P	L	E	G	I	C	■	C	O	N	D	Y	L	■	O
U	N	D	E	R	■	■	X	R	A	Y	■	A	■	E	■	■	A	R
I	■	■	S	H	O	P	■	■	E	■	T	E	N	E	C	T	O	M	Y
V	■	C	A	L	C	A	N	E	O	■	■	A	■	K	■	■	P	■
E	M	E	R	G	E	■	T	■	N	S	A	I	D	■	■	M	■	■	C
R	■	P	I	E	■	F	E	A	S	T	■	A	A	■	M	Y	E	L	O
■	R	I	B	■	I	■	L	I	T	E	■	S	■	■	O	■	■	L
T	■	E	■	S	C	O	L	I	O	S	I	S	■	S	■	■	O
H	C	T	■	C	■	■	C	B	■	S	T	E	N	O	S	I	S
O	■	■	P	■	H	■	A	N	K	L	E	■	E	■	O	■	T
R	O	T	A	T	I	O	N	■	A	■	R	U	B	O	R	■	O
I	■	W	I	■	R	O	D	■	S	■	N	■	M	A	M	M
C	H	O	N	D	R	O	■	A	R	T	H	R	O	G	R	A	P	H	Y

CHAPTER 11–GENITOURINARY SYSTEM

■ Answer Key

The completed crossword grid contains the following answers:

Across/Down entries	
BULBOURETHRAL	NEPHRO
LIRRHAGIA	OLER UV
OPTIC ITIS	CV OSTE
OH H N F	CHAIRS NS
OD OLIGO	S V T S
D BPH	EVALUATE E
GLUCO O E	ME T EU
ENE R ENURESIS	LOOSER R
N PYELONEPHRITIS	I
E RP CD	O C M P N
SCOT UTI	P U PLASIA R
I ON	L E I R
SUTURE GENITOURINARY	

CHAPTER 12–FEMALE REPRODUCTIVE SYSTEM

■ Answer Key

R	E	P	R	O	D	U	C	T	I	V	E		S	A	L	P	I	N	G
A	D	E	N	O		N	E	O		E	A	R	T	H	E	N			R
D	E	N		P	O	I	S	O	N		N		N		E	T			A
I	N	S		H		T	A	L	E	N	T	E	D		P	E	L	V	
O			P	O	S	E	R		C			E			R	B	I		
	F		U	R	O		E		K		B	M			N		D		
F	A	L	L	O	P	I	A	N		P	R	I	M	I	P	A	R	A	
I	T	I	S		H		N	E	P	H	R	O		E		L			
B		M	E	S		T		N		N					M	E			
R		I		M		U		O	N	Y	C	H	O	L	Y	S	I	S	
O	P	T	I	C	I	A	N		S		H		O	A	T	S			
I		C	A	N	D	I	D	I	A	S	I	S		K	G		E		
D	Y	S	U	R	I	A		O	S	T	E	O	P	O	R	O	S	I	S

CHAPTER 13–ENDOCRINE SYSTEM

■ Answer Key

A	L	D	O	S	T	E	R	O	N	E		S	W	E	L	L	I	N	G
D	I		Q		E		N		A	H	O	Y							A
R	P		C	U	T	A	N	E		D	I	M	M	E	R				N
E		N	O	A	H		X		O		T		P		A	B	A		
N	C		M	I	C	R	O	S	C	O	P	E		H	O	P	E	D	
O	O	P	H	O	R		O	R		I			O	R	T	H	O		
	R		S	C	A	N	N	I	N	G		G	M			I			
O	T	O	G	T	O		O	N			E	A	T	I	N	G			
L	E	F	T	Y		L	A	N	G	E	R	H	A	N	S		L	D	L
D	X		N		N		R		D				E		A				
E		O	P	E	N	E	D		A	R		E		G	R	O	I	N	
S		R		C		R	A	P	I	D		N		N			D		
T	H	Y	R	O	I	D	O		H	O	M	E	O	S	T	A	S	I	S

CHAPTER 14–NERVOUS SYSTEM

■ Answer Key

	¹A	²R	³R	⁴H	Y	⁵T	H	⁶M	⁷I	⁸A	S		⁹K	I	¹⁰N	E	S	¹¹I	¹²A	¹³A
	¹⁴M	E	O	W			O		¹⁵N	F	L		E		E			¹⁶T	A	P
¹⁷N	U	M	B	N	¹⁸E	S	S			¹⁹F	O	²⁰U	R		²¹S	L	O	S	H
A				R		T		²²R	E	W	R	A	P	S		²³M	I	A	
²⁴A	²⁵C	²⁶R	O		²⁷N	²⁸S			R		²⁹E	T			³⁰M	A	S	S	
		³¹A	N	³²T	I	E	P	³³I	³⁴L	E	P	T	I	³⁵C	S		C		I
³⁷K	I	T	C	H	E	N		³⁸R	E	N		³⁹E	T	N	A		H		A
N		⁴⁰S	E	A			⁴¹S	H	A	T	T	E	R	I	N	G			
E				L		⁴⁵E		H					S		⁴²I	N	⁴³T	E	R
E		⁴⁴N		⁴⁵A	U	S	⁴⁶T	R	A	L	I	⁴⁷A				T		I	
⁴⁸C	R	E	A	M			A		R			L			⁴⁹T	A	C	H	Y
A			⁵⁰U	⁵¹G	⁵²L	Y		⁵³G	L	⁵⁴I	O	⁵⁵A							
⁵⁶P	A	R	E	S	I	S		⁵⁷H	Y	P	O	T	H	A	L	A	M	U	S

CHAPTER 15–SPECIAL SENSES

■ **Answer Key**

1	2	3	4	5	6	7	8	9	10		11		12		13		14		
H	Y	P	E	R	T	R	O	P	I	A	▓	B	L	E	P	H	A	R	O
E	A	R	D	R	U	M	▓	T	H	U	M	B	▓	A	▓	U	▓		P
A	R	E	▓	H	R	▓	O	D	▓	R	E	T	I	N	A	S			I
R	N	S	▓	E	N	M	E	S	H	I	N	G	▓	C	▓	T			I
I	▓	B	R	A	I	N	▓	I	▓	T	▓	E	S	T	H	E	S	I	A
N	▓	Y	▓	N	▓	S	M	O	O	T	H	▓	U	▓	S	▓			
G	T	O	▓	U	G	L	Y	▓	E	R	▓	E	▓	A	▓	E	O	M	
▓	E	P	I	▓	A	▓	N	Y	S	T	A	G	M	U	S	▓			I
O	S	I	S	▓	B	▓	I	▓	P	▓	R	▓	U	▓	P	R	O		
P	T	A	▓	P	R	I	N	C	E	▓	I	A	S	I	S	▓			T
T	▓	▓	O	▓	O	▓	R	▓	N	▓	▓	I	S	C	H	I			
I	R	I	D	O	▓	S	C	L	E	R	A	▓	G	E	N	▓	Y	▓	C
C	A	T	A	R	A	C	T	▓	S	A	L	P	I	N	G	I	T	I	S

Textbook Medical Record Pronunciations and Answer Key

■ ■ ■ **Chapter 4 – Body Structure**

Medical Record Activity 4–1

Radiological Consultation Letter: Cervical and Lumbar Spine

Terminology

Term	Definition
AP	Abbreviation for *anteroposterior*
atlantoaxial ăt-lăn-tō-ĂK-sē-ăl	Pertaining to the atlas (first cervical vertebra) and the axis (second cervical vertebra)
cervical SĔR-vĭ-kăl	Pertaining to the neck
lateral LĂT-ĕr-ăl	Pertaining to a side
lumbar LŬM-băr	Part of the back between the thorax and pelvis; pertaining to the loins
lumbosacral junction lŭm-bō-SĀ-krăl	Pertaining to the site where the lumbar vertebrae and the sacrum meet
odontoid ō-DŎN-toyd	Toothlike
sacral SĀ-krăl	Pertaining to the sacrum, which is the triangular bone at the base of the spine
scoliosis skō-lē-Ō-sĭs	Lateral curvature of the spine
spasm SPĂZM	Involuntary contraction
spina bifida occulta SPĪ-nă BĬF-ĭ-dă ŏ-KŬL-tă	Failure of the vertebrae to close without hernial protrusion
vertebral bodies VĔR-tĕ-brăl	Pertaining to the large flat, disk-shaped portion of vertebrae

Medical Record Activity 4–2

Radiology Report: Injury of Left Wrist, Elbow, and Humerus

Terminology

Term	Definition
anterior	Pertaining to the front or, in anatomical nomenclature, the *ventral* or *abdominal* side of the body
AP	Anteroposterior
distal DĬS-tăl	Pertaining to the place farthest from the center, medial line, or trunk
dorsal DOR-săl	Pertaining to the back or indicating a position toward a rear part
epicondyle ĕp-ĭ-KŎN-dĭl	Eminence at the articular end of a bone above a condyle
humerus HŪ-mĕr-ŭs	Upper bone of the arm from the elbow to the shoulder joint
lucency LOO-sĕnt-sē	Having the characteristic of being transparent
medial MĒ-dē-ăl	Pertaining to the center
mm	Millimeter (1/1,000 of a meter)
posterior	Pertaining to the back; in anatomical nomenclature, the *dorsal* side of the body
radius RĀ-dē-ŭs	Outer and shorter bone of the forearm on the same side as the thumb
ulna ŬL-nă	Inner and larger bone of the forearm between the wrist and the elbow
ventral-lateral VĔN-trăl-LĂT-ĕr-ăl	Positioned between the front and the side

■ ■ ■ Chapter 5–Integumentary System

Medical Record Activity 5–1

Pathology Report: Skin Lesion

Terminology

Term	Definition
atypia ā-TĬP-ē-ă	State of not being typical
atypical ā-TĬP-ĭ-kăl	Pertaining to tissue that does not show typical characteristics
basal cell layer BĀ-săl	Layer of the epidermis where new cells are formed
Bowen disease BŌ-ĕn dĭ-ZĒZ	Form of intraepidermal carcinoma (squamous cell) characterized by red-brown scaly or crusted lesions that resemble a patch of psoriasis or dermatitis
carcinoma kăr-sĭ-NŌ-mă	New growth or malignant tumor that occurs in epithelial tissue and may infiltrate local tissues or produce metastases
dermatitis dĕr-mă-TĬ-tĭs	Inflammation of the skin
dermis DĔR-mĭs	Layer of skin lying immediately under the epidermis
dorsum DOR-sŭm	Back side of an organ or structure
epidermal hyperplasia ĕp-ĭ-DĔR-măl hī-pĕr-PLĀ-zē-ă	Excessive proliferation of normal cells of the epidermis
fibroplasia fī-brō-PLĀ-sē-ă	Development of fibrous tissue, as in wound healing or by other stimulating factors
hyperkeratosis hī-pĕr-kĕr-ă-TŌ-sĭs	Overgrowth of the horny layer of the epidermis
infiltrate ĬN-fĭl-trāt	To pass into or through a substance or a space
keratinocytes kĕ-RĂT-ĭ-nō-sīts	Any of the cells of the skin that produce keratin
lymphocytic lĭm-fō-SĬT-ĭk	Pertaining to lymphocytes
neoplastic nē-ō-PLĂS-tĭk	Pertaining to any new growth or formation of tissue
papillary PĂP-ĭ-lăr-ē	Pertaining to the layer of the corium that adjoins the epidermis
pathological păth-ō-LŎJ-ĭk-ăl	Pertaining to a diseased condition
solar elastosis SŌ-lăr ĕ-lăs-TŌ-sĭs	Degeneration of collagen fibers as a result of exposure to the sun
squamous SKWĀ-mŭs	Pertaining to or resembling a fish scale

Medical Record Activity 5–2

Patient Referral Letter: Onychomycosis

Terminology

Term	Definition
alkaline phosphatase ĂL-kă-lĭn FŎS-fă-tās	Laboratory test that is a nonspecific indicator of liver disease, bone disease, or hyperparathyroidism
bilaterally bī-LĂT-ĕr-ăl-ē	Pertaining to two sides
CA	Cancer
debridement dā-brēd-MŎN	Removal of foreign material and dead or damaged tissue, especially in a wound; used to promote healing and prevent infection
hypertension hī-pĕr-TĔN-shŭn	Condition that is present when, on several separate occasions, blood pressure in an adult registers 140/90 or higher (The optimal pressure is 120/80.)
mastectomy măs-TĔK-tŏ-mē	Surgical excision of a breast
neurological noor-ō-LŎJ-ĭk-ăl	Pertaining to a nerve or nervous tissue
onychomycosis ŏn-ĭ-kō-mī-KŌ-sĭs	Fungal infection of the nail or nail bed
Sporanox SPOR-ă-nŏks	Trade name for itraconazole
vascular VĂS-kū-lăr	Pertaining to a blood vessel

■ ■ ■ Chapter 6–Digestive System

Medical Record Activity 6–1

Chart Note: GI Evaluation

Terminology

Term	Definition
appendectomy ăp-ĕn-DĔK-tō-mē	Removal of the appendix
cholecystectomy kō-lē-sĭs-TĔK-tō-mē	Removal of the gallbladder
cholecystitis kō-lē-sĭs-TĪ-tĭs	Inflammation of the gallbladder
cholelithiasis kō-lē-lĭ-THĪ-ă-sĭs	Presence or formation of gallstones

Term	Definition
crescendo kră-SHĔN-dō	Gradually increasing in intensity or strength
decrescendo dā-kră-SHĔN-dō	Gradually decreasing in intensity or strength
defecate DĔF-ĕ-kāt	Evacuate the bowels; bowel movement
flatus FLĀ-tŭs	Expelling of gas from a body orifice, especially the anus
heme-negative stool hēm-NĔG-ă-tĭv	Stool that shows a negative result for the presence of occult blood
hepatomegaly hĕp-ă-tō-MĔG-ă-lē	Enlargement of the liver
intermittent ĭn-tĕr-MĬT-ĕnt	Suspending activity at intervals; coming and going
nausea NAW-sē-ă	Unpleasant, wavelike sensation in the back of the throat, epigastrium, or throughout the abdomen that may or may not lead to vomiting
PMH	Past medical history
postoperative pōst-ŎP-ĕr-ă-tĭv	Occurring after surgery
R/O	Rule out
splenomegaly splē-nō-MĔG-ă-lē	Enlargement of the spleen
tonsillectomy tŏn-sĭl-ĔK-tō-mē	Removal of the tonsils

Medical Record Activity 6–2

Operative Report: Esophagogastroduodenoscopy with Biopsy

Terminology

Term	Definition
Demerol DĔM-ĕr-ŏl	Trade name for an opiate analgesic used to treat moderate to severe pain
duodenal bulb dū-ō-DĒ-năl BŬLB	First portion of the duodenum; also called *duodenal cap*
duodenitis dū-ŏd-ĕ-NĪ-tĭs	Inflammation of the duodenum
erythema ĕr-ĭ-THĒ-mă	Redness of the skin produced by congestion of the capillaries
esophageal varices ē-sŏf-ă-JĒ-ăl VĂR-ĭ-sēz	Varicose veins of the esophagus

Term	Definition
esophagogastroduodenoscopy ĕ-sŏf-ă-gō-găs-trō-doo-ŏ-dĕn-ŎS-kō-pē	Inspection of the esophagus, stomach, and duodenum using an endoscope
etiology ē-tē-ŎL-ō-jē	Study of the causes of a disease
friability frī-ă-BĬL-ĭ-tē	Ability to be easily broken or pulverized
gastric antrum GĂS-trĭk ĂN-trŭm	Portion of the stomach immediately before the outlet that is lined by mucosa but does not produce acid
gastritis găs-TRĪ-tĭs	Inflammation of the stomach
hematemesis hĕm-ăt-ĔM-ĕ-sĭs	Vomiting of blood
lateral recumbent LĂT-ĕr-ăl rē-KŬM-bĕnt	Lying or reclining on the side
oximeter ŏk-SĬM-ĕ-tĕr	Instrument that measures the amount of oxygen in blood
punctate erythema PŬNK-tāt ĕr-ĭ-THĒ-mă	Redness of the skin in the form of tiny red dots
tomography tō-MŎG-ră-fē	Imaging technique achieved by rotating an x-ray emitter around the area to be scanned and measuring the intensity of transmitted rays from different angles
Versed VĔR-sĕd	CNS depressant with sedative, muscle relaxant, anticonvulsant, and amnesiac effects
videoendoscope vĭd-ē-ō-ĔND-ō-skōp	Endoscope fitted with a device that allows projection of images on a video monitor

■ ■ ■ Chapter 7–Respiratory System

Medical Record Activity 7–1

SOAP Note: Respiratory Evaluation

Terminology

Term	Definition
anteriorly ăn-TĒR-ē-or-lē	Pertaining to the front or, in anatomical nomenclature, the *ventral* or *abdominal* side of the body
bilateral bī-LĂT-ĕr-ăl	Pertaining to or relating to two sides
COPD	Chronic obstructive pulmonary disease
exacerbation ĕks-ăs-ĕr-BĀ-shŭn	Increase in the severity of a disease or disorder as marked by greater intensity in the patient's signs or symptoms

Term	Definition
heart failure	Condition in which the heart fails to pump an adequate supply of blood to meet the needs of the body
Hx	History
hypertension hī-pĕr-TĔN-shŭn	Persistently elevated arterial blood pressure
interstitial ĭn-tĕr-STĬSH-ăl	Pertaining to the spaces between the cells of tissues
PE	Physical examination
peripheral vascular disease pĕr-ĬF-ĕr-ăl VĂS-kū-lăr dĭ-ZĒZ	Any disease of the blood vessels that lie outside the heart
pleural PLOO-răl	Pertaining to the pleura (double-folded membrane covering the lungs)
posteriorly pŏs-TĒR-ē-or-lē	Pertaining to the back or, in anatomical nomenclature, the *dorsal* side of the body
rhonchi RŎNG-kī	Rattling sound heard in breathing due to obstruction in the air passages
SOB	Shortness of breath
wheezes HWĒZ-ĕz	Continuous musical sound caused by the narrowing of the lumen of the respiratory structures

Medical Record Activity 7–2

SOAP Note: Chronic Interstitial Lung Disease

Terminology

Term	Definition
ABG	Arterial blood gas
adenopathy ăd-ĕ-NŎP-ă-thē	Disease of a gland
basilar crackles BĂS-ĭ-lăr KRĂK-ĕlz	Sharp or scratchy sound originating from the base of the lungs (basilar) heard with a stethoscope and commonly associated with pleurisy
cardiomyopathy kăr-dē-ō-mī-ŎP-ă-thē	Any disease of the heart muscle
chronic KRŎN-ĭk	Persisting over a long period of time
diuresis dī-ū-RĒ-sĭs	Increase in the production of urine
dyspnea dĭsp-NĒ-ă	Difficulty breathing
fibrosis fī-BRŌ-sĭs	Repair and replacement of inflamed tissues or organs with connective tissues

Term	Definition
interstitial ĭn-tĕr-STĬSH-ăl	Pertaining to the spaces between the cells of tissues
kyphosis kī-FŌ-sĭs	Exaggeration or angulation of the normal posterior curve of the spine, causing the condition commonly know as *humpback, hunchback,* or *Pott curvature*
Lasix LĀ-sĭks	Diuretic medication (furosemide) used to promote excretion of urine
neuropathy nū-RŎP-ă-thē	Any disease of a nerve
PCO₂	Partial pressure of carbon dioxide
pedal edema PĔD-lĕ-DĒ-mă	Edema or swelling of the feet
pH	Symbol for degree of acidity or alkalinity
PO₂	Partial pressure of oxygen
pulmonary fibrosis PŬL-mō-nĕ-rē fī-BRŌ-sĭs	Replacement of inflamed pulmonary tissue with connective tissue
renal insufficiency RĒ-năl ĭn-sŭ-FĬSH-ĕn-sē	Inadequate kidney function
rhonchi RŎNG-kī	Rattling sound heard during breathing caused by obstruction in the air passages
silicosis sĭl-ĭ-KŌ-sĭs	Inflammation and scarring of lungs from inhalation of silica dust (glass or sand)
thyromegaly thī-rō-MĔG-ă-lē	Enlargement of the thyroid

■ ■ ■ Chapter 8–Cardiovascular System

Medical Record Activity 8–1

Chart Note: Acute Myocardial Infarction

Terminology

Term	Definition
acute	Having a rapid onset, severe symptoms, and a short course
cardiac enzymes KĂR-dē-ăk ĔN-zīmz	Protein molecules released into the blood stream from heart muscle damaged by a blocked artery
CCU	Coronary care unit
ECG	Electrocardiogram; electrocardiograph
heparin HĔP-ă-rĭn	Agent that inhibits or stops blood from clotting
infarction ĭn-FĂRK-shŭn	Death of tissue that results from deprivation of its blood supply

Term	Definition
inferior	Beneath or lower and used medically in reference to the undersurface of an organ or indicating a structure below another structure
ischemia ĭs-KĒ-mē-ă	Temporary deficiency of blood flow to an organ or tissue
lateral LĂT-ĕr-ăl	Pertaining or relating to a side
MI	Myocardial infarction
myocardial mī-ō-KĂR-dē-ăl	Pertaining to the heart muscle
partial thromboplastin time thrŏm-bō-PLĂS-tĭn	Laboratory test that measures the intrinsic clotting time in plasma
streptokinase strĕp-tō-KĪ-nās	Agent that destroys or dissolves blood clots
substernal sŭb-STĔR-năl	Pertaining to the area below the sternum

Medical Record Activity 8–2

Operative Report: Right Temporal Artery Biopsy

Terminology

Term	Definition
arteritis ăr-tĕ-RĪ-tĭs	Inflammation of an artery
Betadine BĀ-tă-dīn	Trade name for an iodine-containing topical antiseptic agent
biopsy BĪ-ŏp-sē	Representative tissue sample removed from a body site for microscopic examination, usually to establish a diagnosis
dissected dī-SĔKT-ĕd	Cut to separate and study a part
distally DĬS-tă-lē	Pertaining to the place farthest from the center, medial line, or trunk
incised ĭn-SĪZD	Cut into
IV	Intravenous
ligated LĪ-gā-tĕd	Applied a binding or suture for tying of a blood vessel or other structure
palpable PĂL-pă-b'l	Perceptible by touch
preauricular prē-aw-RĬK-ū-lăr	Pertaining to the area in front of the ear

Term	Definition
proximally PRŎK-sĭ-mă-lē	Nearest the point of attachment, center of the body, or point of reference
superficial fascia soo-pĕr-FĬSH-ăl FĂSH-ē-ă	Fibrous membrane covering, supporting, and separating muscles
supine sū-PĪN	Lying on the back
temporal TĔM-por-ăl	Pertaining to the temples
Xylocaine ZĪ-lō-kān	Trade name for a local skin anesthetic

■ ■ ■ Chapter 9–Blood, Lymph, and Immune System

Medical Record Activity 9–1

Discharge Summary: Sickle Cell Crisis

Terminology

Term	Definition
ambulating ĂM-bū-lāt-ĭng	Walking
analgesia ăn-ăl-JĒ-zē-ă	Absence of a normal sense of pain
anemia ă-NĒ-mē-ă	Reduction in the mass of circulating red blood cells
crisis KRĪ-sĭs	Turning point of a disease, which is a critical period commonly marked by a long sleep and profuse perspiration
CT scan	Computed tomography scan
hemoglobin HĒ-mō-glō-bĭn	Iron-containing pigment of red blood cells that carries oxygen from the lungs to the tissues
ileus ĬL-ē-ŭs	Intestinal obstruction
infarction ĭn-FĂRK-shŭn	Tissue death that results from deprivation of blood supply
morphine MOR-fēn	Principal alkaloid found in opium, occurring as bitter, colorless crystals, and commonly used in oral or injectable form to control severe, acute, or chronic pain
sickle cell SĬK-ăl SĔL	Abnormal erythrocyte that appears as a club or sickle shape due to an abnormal form of hemoglobin (HgbS)
splenectomy splē-NĔK-tō-mē	Excision of the spleen
Vicodin VĪ-kō-dĭn	Trade name for a combination of a narcotic analgesic (painkiller) and cough reliever with a nonnarcotic analgesic for the relief of moderate to moderately severe pain

Medical Record Activity 9–2

Discharge Summary: PCP and HIV

Terminology

Term	Definition
alveolar lavage ăl-VĒ-ō-lăr lă-VĂZH	Washing of the lower respiratory tract with saline to collect specimens for analysis
Bactrim BĂK-trĭm	Trade name for an antibiotic commonly prescribed for *Pneumocystis* pneumonia and prevention of this type of pneumonia in people with weakened immune systems
bronchoscopy brŏng-KŎS-kō-pē	Visual examination of the interior tracheobronchial tree through a bronchoscope
diffuse dĭ-FŪS	Spreading or scattered
HIV	Human immunodeficiency virus
human immunodeficiency virus ĭm-ū-nō-dē-FĬSH-ĕn-sē	Causative organism of acquired immune deficiency syndrome; a virus that attacks the immune system
infiltrate ĬN-fĭl-trāt	To pass into or through a substance or space
Kaposi sarcoma KĂP-ō-sē săr-KŌ-mă	Malignancy that develops in connective tissues, such as cartilage, bone, fat, muscle, blood vessels, and fibrous tissues (related to tendons or ligaments) and is commonly associated with HIV infection
leukoencephalopathy loo-kō-ĕn-sĕf-ă-LŎP-ă-thē	Rare disorder of the nervous system characterized by demyelination or destruction of the myelin sheath that covers nerve cells and primarily affects individuals with suppressed immune systems
multifocal mŭl-tĭ-FŌ-kăl	Pertining to or arising from many locations
PCP	*Pneumocystis* pneumonia
PMN	Polymorphonuclear leukocyte
***Pneumocystis* pneumonia** nū-mō-SĬS-tĭs kă-RĪ-nē-ī nū-MŌ-nē-ă	Pneumonia caused by the *Pneumocystis* organism
thrush THRŬSH	Fungal infection of the mucosa of the mouth caused by the *Candida albicans* organism
vaginal candidiasis VĂJ-ĭn-ăl kăn-dĭ-DĪ-ă-sĭs	Fungal infection of the vagina caused by the *Candida albicans* organism

■ ■ ■ Chapter 10–Musculoskeletal System

Medical Record Activity 10–1

**Operative Report: Right Knee Arthroscopy
and Medial Meniscectomy**

Terminology

Term	Definition
ACL	Anterior cruciate ligament
arthroscopy ăr-THRŎS-kō-pē	Examination of a joint using a specialized endoscope
effusions ĕ-FŪ-zhŭnz	Escape of fluids into a body part or body tissue
intracondylar ĭn-tră-KŎN-dĭ-lăr	Pertaining to the area within the rounded surface at the extremity of a bone
Lachman test LĂK-măn	Maneuver to detect deficiency of the anterior cruciate ligament in which the knee is flexed at 30 degrees and the tibia is displaced anteriorly relative to the femur (A soft endpoint or displacement greater than 4 mm is positive, or abnormal.)
McMurray sign test	Test for a torn meniscus of the knee
meniscectomy mĕn-ĭ-SĔK-tō-mē	Removal of the meniscus cartilage of the knee
MRI	Magnetic resonance imaging
PCL	Posterior cruciate ligament
synovitis sĭn-ō-VĪ-tĭs	Inflammation of the synovial membrane of a joint

Medical Record Activity 10–2

**Radiographic Consultation: Tibial Diaphysis
Nuclear Scan**

Terminology

Term	Definition
buttressing BŬT-rĕs-ĭng	Supporting or reinforcing another structure
cortical KOR-tĭ-kăl	Pertaining to the outer coat of a structure
diaphysis dī-ĂF-ĭ-sĭs	Shaft or middle part of a long cylindrical bone
endosteal ĕn-DŎS-tē-ăl	Pertaining to the membrane that lines the marrow cavity of a bone

Term	Definition
focal FŌ-kăl	Pertaining to the starting point of a disease process
fusiform FŪ-zĭ-form	Tapering at both ends; spindle-shaped
NSAIDs	Nonsteroidal anti-inflammatory drugs
nuclear scan NŪ-klē-ăr	Diagnostic technique that uses a radioactive material (radiopharmaceutical) introduced into the body (inhaled, ingested, or injected) and a scanning device to determine size, shape, location, and function of various organs and structures
periosteal pĕr-ē-ŎS-tē-ăl	Pertaining to the fibrous membrane that forms the covering of bones except at their articular surfaces
resorption rē-SORP-shŭn	Removal by absorption, as of an exudate or pus
tibial TĬB-ē-ăl	Pertaining to the tibia, the inner and larger bone of the leg between the knee and ankle

■ ■ ■ Chapter 11–Genitourinary System

Medical Record Activity 11–1

Operative Report: Ureterocele and Ureterocele Calculus

Terminology

Term	Definition
calculus KĂL-kū-lŭs	Solid concretion or stone that forms in the urinary tract
cystolithotripsy sĭs-tō-LĬTH-ō-trĭp-sē	Crushing of a stone in the urinary bladder
cystoscope SĬST-ō-skōp	Endoscope used to examine the bladder
fulguration fŭl-gŭ-RĀ-shŭn	Destruction of tissue by means of long, high-frequency electric sparks
hematuria hē-mă-TŪ-rē-ă	Blood in the urine
resectoscope rē-SĔK-tō-skōp	Instrument for removing the prostate gland through the urethra
transurethral trăns-ū-RĒ-thrăl	Pertaining to a procedure preformed through the urethra
ureterocele ū-RĒ-tĕr-ō-sēl	Prolapse or herniation of the terminal part of the ureter into the bladder
urethral sound ū-RĒ-thrăl	Instrument used to dilate the urethra

Medical Record Activity 11-2

Operative Report: Extracorporeal Shockwave Lithotripsy

Terminology

Term	Definition
calculus KĂL-kū-lŭs	Solid concretion or stone that forms in the urinary tract
calyx KĀ-lĭx	Cuplike organ or cavity
cystoscope SĬST-ō-skōp	Endoscope used to examine the bladder
cystoscopy sĭs-TŎS-kō-pē	Examination of the bladder using a specialized endoscope
dorsal lithotomy DOR-săl lĭth-ŎT-ō-mē	Lying or reclining on the side
ESWL	Extracorporeal shockwave lithotripsy
extracorporeal ĕks-tră-kor-POR-ē-ăl	Pertaining to the outside of the body
fluoroscopy floo-or-ŎS-kō-pē	Radiographic technique in which x-rays are directed through the body to a fluorescent screen that displays continuous imaging of the motion of internal structures and immediate serial images
lithotripsy LĬTH-ō-trĭp-sē	Crushing of a stone
shock wave	Powerful sound wave that causes vibrations used to break up calculi in the urinary tract or gallbladder
staghorn calculus STĂG-horn KĂL-kū-lŭs	Renal stone that develops in the renal pelvis and, in advanced cases, has a branching configuration that resembles the antlers of a stag
stent stĕnt	Small rod or threadlike device used to support tubular structures during surgical anastomosis or hold arteries open during angioplasty

■ ■ ■ Chapter 12–Female Reproductive System

Medical Record Activity 12–1

SOAP Note: Primary Herpes 1 Infection

Terminology

Term	Definition
adenopathy ăd-ĕ-NŎP-ă-thē	Swelling and morbid change in lymph nodes; glandular disease
chlamydia klă-MĬD-ē-ă	Sexually transmitted disease responsible for most cases of cervicitis in women and urethritis, proctitis, and pharyngitis in both sexes

Term	Definition
GC screen	Gonococcal screen
herpes lesions HĔR-pēz LĒ-zhŭnz	Small clusters of painful vesicles that generally become crusted and heal in about 10 days and are symptomatic of herpes infection
introitus īn-TRŌ-ĭ-tŭs	Opening or entrance into a canal or cavity, such as the vagina
labia LĀ-bē-ă	Two pairs of skin and adipose tissue (labia majora and labia minora) that lie at the entrance of the vagina
LMP	Last menstrual period
monilial mō-NĬL-ē-ăl	Pertaining to monilia, a fungal organism responsible for common infections usually occuring in the mouth or vagina; more commonly called *candida*
OCPs	Oral contraceptive pills
pruritus proo-RĪ-tŭs	Extreme itching
R/O	Rule out
vulvar VŬL-văr	Pertaining to the vulva, the external female genitalia
Wet prep WĔT PRĔP	Technique used to identify various causes of vaginitis, by applying a specimen to a slide containing either saline or potassium hydroxide, and examining it using a microscope

Medical Record Activity 12–2

Preoperative Consultation: Menometrorrhagia

Terminology

Term	Definition
ablation ăb-LĀ-shŭn	Removal of a part, pathway, or function by surgery, chemical destruction, electrocautery, or radiofrequency
benign bē-NĪN	Not recurrent or progressive; also called *nonmalignant*
cesarean section sē-SĀR-ē-ăn	Delivery of a fetus by means of an incision into the uterus
cholecystectomy kō-lē-sĭs-TĔK-tō-mē	Removal of the gallbladder
dysmenorrhea dĭs-mĕn-ō-RĒ-ă	Pain associated with menstruation
endometrial biopsy ĕn-dō-MĒ-trē-ăl BĪ-ŏp-sē	Removal of a small sample of tissue from the endometrium for examination
fibroids FĪ-broyds	Benign tumors of the uterine myometrium
gravida 2 GRĂV-ĭ-dă	Term indicating a woman who has been pregnant two times

Term	Definition
hysterectomy hĭs-tĕr-ĔK-tō-mē	Surgical removal of the uterus
laparoscopic lăp-ă-rō-SKŎP-ĭk	Pertaining to an abdominal exploration of the inner surface of the uterus with a specially designed endoscope called a *laparoscope*
mammogram MĂM-ō-grăm	X-ray image of the breast
menometrorrhagia mĕn-ō-mĕt-rō-RĀ-jē-ă	Excessive bleeding during and between menstrual periods
palliative PĂL-ē-ā-tĭv	Relieving or alleviating without curing
para 1 PĂR-ă	Woman who has given birth to one viable fetus
postoperative pōst-ŎP-ĕr-ă-tĭv	Time after surgery
Premarin PRĔM-ă-rĭn	Agent used to treat adverse symptoms of menopause, including hot flashes, vaginal dryness, and fatigue, through hormone replacement therapy (HRT)
salpingo-oophorectomy săl-pĭng-gō-ō-ŏf-ō-RĔK-tō-mē	Surgical removal of the fallopian tubes and ovaries
therapeutic abortion thĕr-ă-PŪ-tĭk ă-BOR-shŭn	Abortion performed for medical reasons
thyroid function test THĪ-royd FŬNG-shŭn	Blood test used to determine disorders of the thyroid that commonly includes determining the concentration of T_3 (thyroxine) and T_4 (triiodothyronine)

■ ■ ■ Chapter 13–Endocrine System

Medical Record Activity 13–1

Consultation Note: Hyperparathyroidism

Terminology

Term	Definition
adenoma ăd-ĕ-NŌ-mă	Benign tumor made of epithelial cells, usually arranged like a gland
claudication klăw-dĭ-KĀ-shŭn	Lameness
diabetes mellitus dī-ă-BĒ-tēz MĔ-lĭ-tŭs	Chronic metabolic disorder marked by hyperglycemia; also called *type 1 diabetes mellitus* or *insulin-dependent diabetes mellitus*
endocrinologist ĕn-dō-krĭn-ŎL-ō-jĭst	Specialist in the treatment of endocrine disorders
hypercalciuria hī-pĕr-kăl-sē-Ū-rē-ă	Excessive calcium levels in urine

Term	Definition
hyperparathyroidism hī-pĕr-păr-ă-THĪ-roy-dĭzm	Condition caused by excessive levels of parathyroid hormone in the body
impression ĭm-PRĔSH-ŭn	Disease or condition the patient is thought to have; also called *diagnosis*
osteoarthritis ŏs-tē-ō-ăr-THRĪ-tĭs	Type of arthritis marked by progressive cartilage deterioration in synovial joints and vertebrae
parathyroid păr-ă-THĪ-royd	One of four small endocrine glands on the back of and at the lower edge of the thyroid gland that secrete parathyroid hormone
peripheral vascular disease pĕr-ĬF-ĕr-ăl VĂS-kū-lăr dĭ-ZĒZ	Progressive occlusive disease that affects the arteries of the extremities

Medical Record Activity 13–2

SOAP Note: Diabetes Mellitus

Terminology

Term	Definition
Accu-chek ĂK-ū-chĕk	Home testing product used to determine blood glucose levels
morbid obesity MOR-bĭd ō-BĒ-sĭ-tē	Body weight more that 100 lb over ideal body weight (IBW)
obesity, exogenous ō-BĒ-sĭ-tē, ĕks-ŎJ-ĕ-nŭs	Obesity caused by overeating
polydipsia pŏl-ē-DĬP-sē-ă	Excessive thirst
polyphagia pŏl-ē-FĀ-jē-ă	Eating abnormally large amounts of food; also known as *gluttony*
polyuria pŏl-ē-Ū-rē-ă	Excessive secretion and discharge of urine

■ ■ ■ Chapter 14–Nervous System

Medical Record Activity 14–1

Discharge Summary: Subarachnoid Hemorrhage

Terminology

Term	Definition
aneurysm ĂN-ū-rĭzm	Localized abnormal dilation of a vessel, usually an artery
cerebral MRI sĕ-RĒ-brăl	Noninvasive imaging technique that uses radio waves and a strong magnetic field, rather than an x-ray beam, to produce multiplanar cross-sectional images of the cerebrum
cisterna subarachnoidalis sĭs-TĔR-nă sŭb-ă-răk-NOYD-ă-lĭs	Cavity or space located beneath the arachnoid containing cerebrospinal fluid
CSF	Cerebrospinal fluid
CT scan	Computed tomography scan
hydrocephalus hī-drō-SĔF-ă-lŭs	Dilation of the ventricle caused by the accumulation of cerebrospinal fluid that has failed to drain properly, resulting in an enlargement of the head
lumbar puncture LŬM-băr PŬNK-chŭr	Introduction of a hollow needle and stylet into the subarachnoid space of the lumbar part of the spinal canal, usually at the level of the fourth intervertebral space, to obtain CSF for analysis
meningismus mĕn-ĭn-JĬS-mŭs	Irritation of the brain and spinal cord with symptoms simulating meningitis but without actual inflammation
occipital ŏk-SĬP-ĭ-tăl	Skull bone positioned between the parietal and temporal bones
R/O	Rule out
subarachnoid sŭb-ă-RĂK-noyd	Space beneath the arachnoid

Medical Record Activity 14–2

Consultation Report: Acute Onset Paraplegia

Terminology

Term	Definition
abscess ĂB-sĕs	Localized collection of pus in any body part that results from invasion of a pyogenic bacterium or other pathogen
acute ă-KŪT	Sharp, severe condition with a rapid onset and a short course
clonidine KLŌ-nĭ-dēn	Centrally acting antihypertensive medication
epidural ĕp-ĭ-DOO-răl	Situated within the spinal canal, on or above the dura mater

Term	Definition
fluoroscopy floo-or-ŎS-kō-pē	Visual examination of a part of the body or the function of an organ using a fluoroscope, which offers continuous imaging of the motion of internal structures and immediate serial images
infarct ĬN-fărkt	Area of tissue in an organ or part that undergoes necrosis following cessation of the blood supply
L2-3	Second and third lumbar vertebrae
lumbar LŬM-băr	Part of the back between the thorax and the pelvis
methadone MĔTH-ă-dōn	Analgesic narcotic used in the management of severe pain
myelitis mī-ě-LĪ-tĭs	Inflammation of the spinal cord
paraplegia păr-ă-PLĒ-jē-ă	Paralysis of the lower body and both legs
paresthesia păr-ĕs-THĒ-zē-ă	Abnormal or unpleasant sensations that result from injury to one or more nerves, commonly described by patients as numbness or as a prickly, stinging, or burning feeling
subarachnoid sŭb-ă-RĂK-noyd	Space beneath the arachnoid
T10-11	Tenth and eleventh thoracic vertebrae
transverse trăns-VĔRS	Lying at right angles to the long axis of the body

■ ■ ■ Chapter 15–Special Senses

Medical Record Activity 15–1

Operative Report: Retained Foreign Bodies

Terminology

Term	Definition
bilateral bī-LĂT-ĕr-ăl	Pertaining to two sides
cerumen sĕ-ROO-mĕn	Earwax
perforation pĕr-fō-RĀ-shŭn	Small hole or opening
supine sū-PĪN	Lying on the back, with face upward
tympanostomy tĭm-pă-NŎS-tō-mē	Incision of the tympanic membrane; also called *myringotomy*

Medical Record Activity 15-2

Operative Report: Phacoemulsification and Lens Implant

Terminology

Term	Definition
anesthesia ăn-ĕs-THĒ-zē-ă	Partial or complete loss of sensation, with or without loss of consciousness, as a result of disease, injury, or administration of an anesthetic agent
blepharostat BLĔF-ă-rō-stăt	Device used to separate the eyelids during surgery
capsulorrhexis kăp-sū-lō-RĔK-sĭs	Common method of cataract extraction in which a circular incision is made in the anterior capsule to permit lens extraction
cataract KĂT-ă-răkt	Opacity of the lens of the eye, usually occurring as a result of aging, trauma, or disease
conjunctival kŏn-jŭnk-TĪ-văl	Pertaining to the conjunctiva
diopter dī-ŎP-tĕr	Metric measure of the refractive power of a lens used as a unit of measurement in refraction
intravenous ĭn-tră-VĒ-nŭs	Within or into a vein
keratome KĔR-ă-tōm	Knife used to incise a cornea; also called *keratotome*
peritomy pĕr-ĬT-ō-mē	Excision of a narrow strip of conjunctiva around the cornea
phacoemulsification fā-kō-ē-mŭl-sĭ-fĭ-KĀ-shŭn	Method of treating a cataract that uses an ultrasonic device to disintegrate the cataract, which is then aspirated and removed
posterior chamber	Space behind the iris but in front of and at the side of the lens
retrobulbar block rĕt-rō-BŬL-băr	Procedure used in surgery on the eye that provides adequate anesthesia, akinesia, and control of intraocular pressure as well as postoperative analgesia
sutures SŪ-chŭrz	Thread of catgut, silk, or wire used to stitch parts of the body together
TobraDex TŌ-bră-dĕks	Trade name for an antibiotic used to treat external ocular infections

Master Transparencies

The following section offers a series of gray-scale images made especially for overhead transparencies.

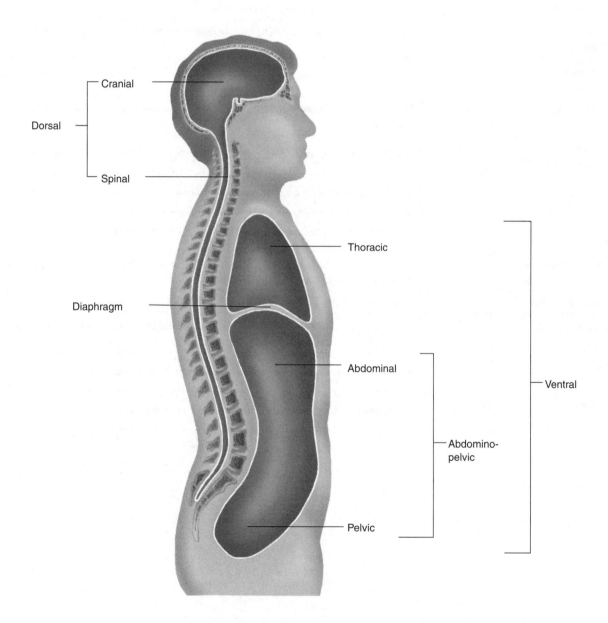

Copyright © 2009. F. A. Davis. *Activity Pack to Accompany Medical Terminology Systems,* 6th ed.

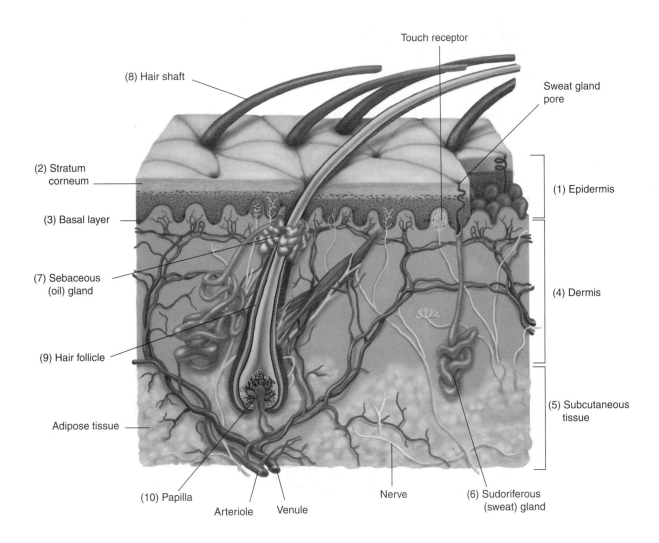

Touch receptor

(8) Hair shaft

Sweat gland pore

(2) Stratum corneum

(1) Epidermis

(3) Basal layer

(7) Sebaceous (oil) gland

(4) Dermis

(9) Hair follicle

Adipose tissue

(5) Subcutaneous tissue

(10) Papilla

Arteriole   Venule

Nerve

(6) Sudoriferous (sweat) gland

A. Inspiration:
  Air drawn into lungs

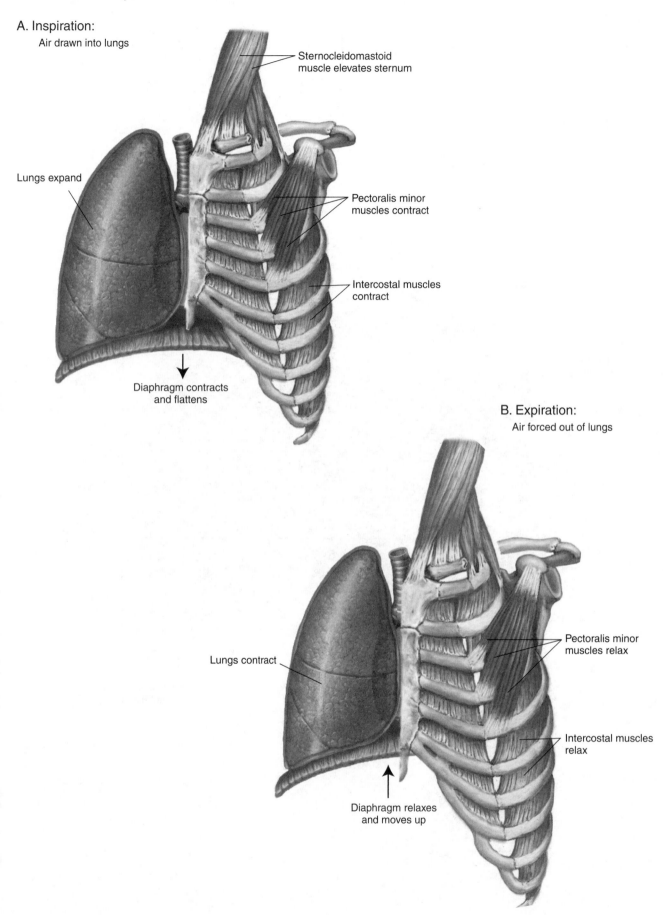

Sternocleidomastoid
muscle elevates sternum

Lungs expand

Pectoralis minor
muscles contract

Intercostal muscles
contract

Diaphragm contracts
and flattens

B. Expiration:
  Air forced out of lungs

Pectoralis minor
muscles relax

Lungs contract

Intercostal muscles
relax

Diaphragm relaxes
and moves up

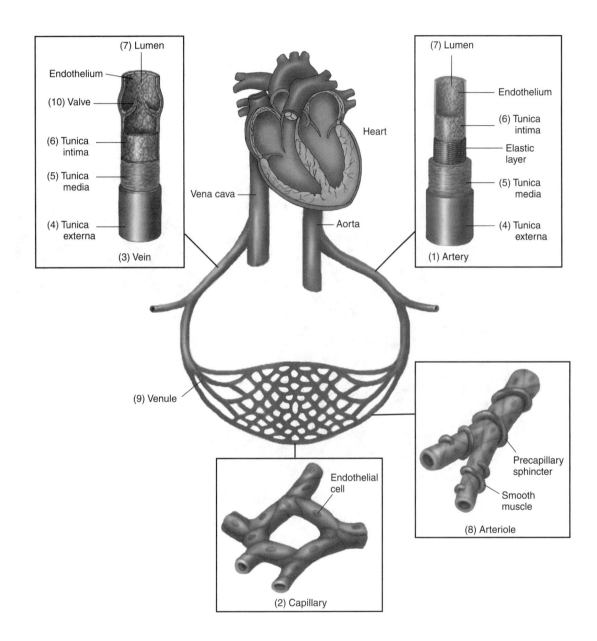

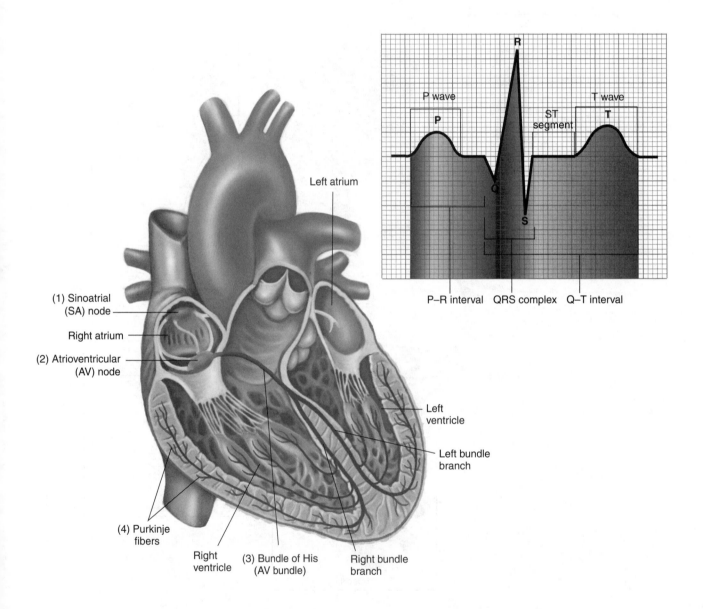

P wave

P

R

ST segment

T wave

T

Q

S

Left atrium

(1) Sinoatrial (SA) node

Right atrium

(2) Atrioventricular (AV) node

Left ventricle

Left bundle branch

(4) Purkinje fibers

Right ventricle

(3) Bundle of His (AV bundle)

Right bundle branch

P–R interval   QRS complex   Q–T interval

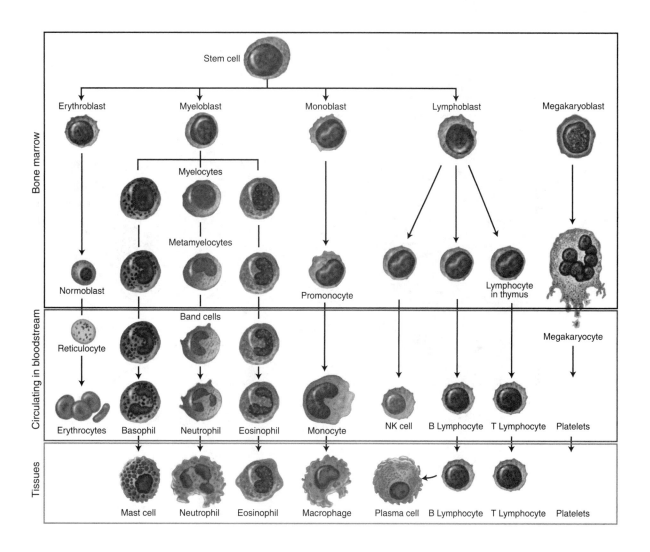

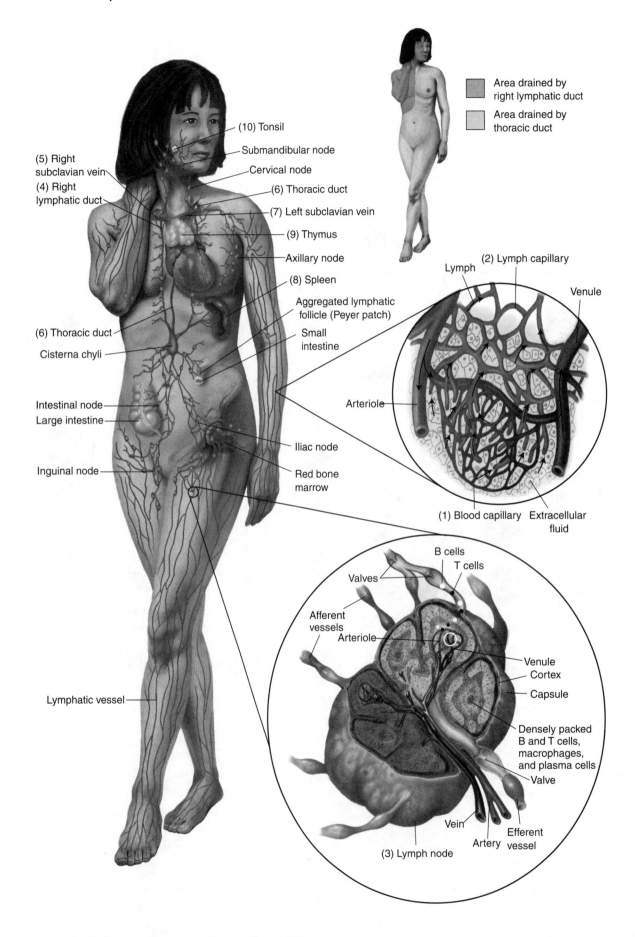

Area drained by
right lymphatic duct

Area drained by
thoracic duct

(10) Tonsil

Submandibular node

Cervical node

(5) Right
subclavian vein

(4) Right
lymphatic duct

(6) Thoracic duct

(7) Left subclavian vein

(9) Thymus

Axillary node

(8) Spleen

Aggregated lymphatic
follicle (Peyer patch)

Small
intestine

(6) Thoracic duct

Cisterna chyli

Intestinal node

Large intestine

Inguinal node

Iliac node

Red bone
marrow

Lymphatic vessel

Lymph

(2) Lymph capillary

Venule

Arteriole

(1) Blood capillary   Extracellular
fluid

B cells

T cells

Valves

Afferent
vessels

Arteriole

Venule

Cortex

Capsule

Densely packed
B and T cells,
macrophages,
and plasma cells

Valve

Vein

Artery

Efferent
vessel

(3) Lymph node

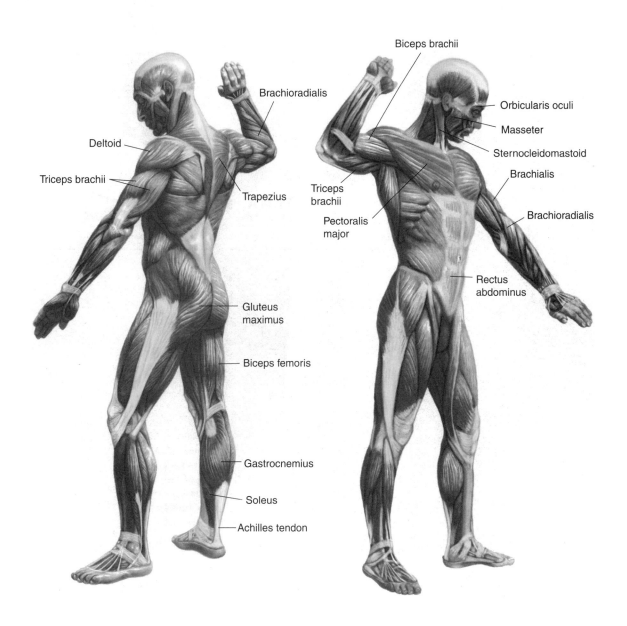

Biceps brachii

Brachioradialis

Deltoid

Triceps brachii

Trapezius

Orbicularis oculi

Masseter

Sternocleidomastoid

Triceps brachii

Brachialis

Pectoralis major

Brachioradialis

Gluteus maximus

Rectus abdominus

Biceps femoris

Gastrocnemius

Soleus

Achilles tendon

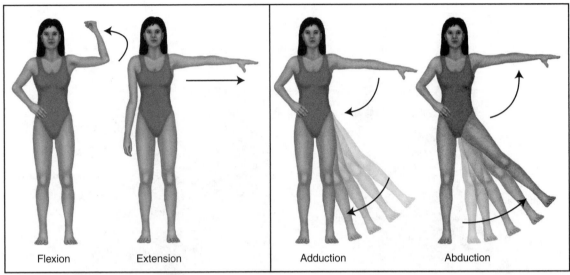

Flexion   Extension   Adduction   Abduction

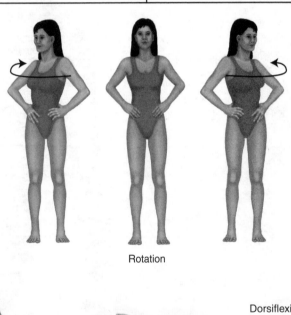

Rotation

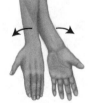

Pronation   Supination

Eversion   Inversion

Dorsiflexion

Plantar flexion

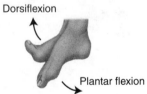

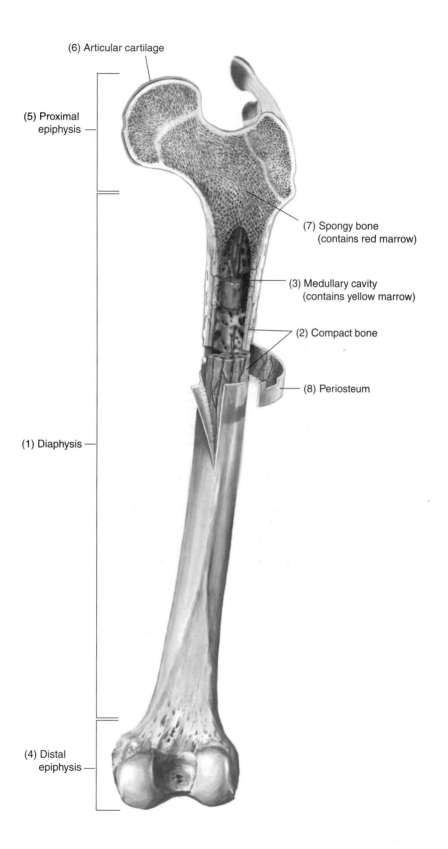

(6) Articular cartilage

(5) Proximal
epiphysis

(7) Spongy bone
(contains red marrow)

(3) Medullary cavity
(contains yellow marrow)

(2) Compact bone

(8) Periosteum

(1) Diaphysis

(4) Distal
epiphysis

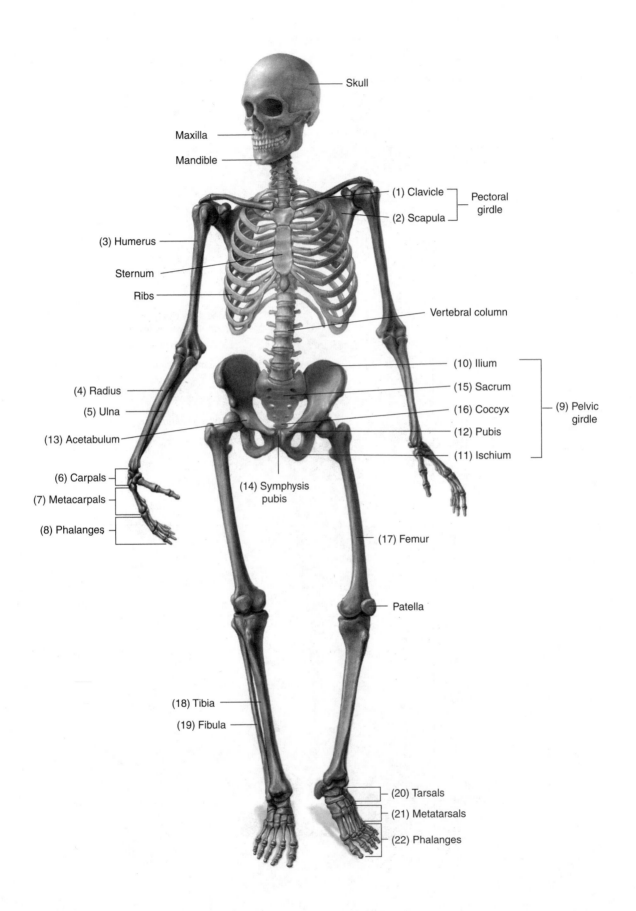

Skull

Maxilla

Mandible

(1) Clavicle
(2) Scapula

Pectoral girdle

(3) Humerus

Sternum

Ribs

Vertebral column

(10) Ilium
(15) Sacrum

(4) Radius
(5) Ulna

(16) Coccyx

(13) Acetabulum

(12) Pubis

(9) Pelvic girdle

(11) Ischium

(6) Carpals

(7) Metacarpals

(8) Phalanges

(14) Symphysis pubis

(17) Femur

Patella

(18) Tibia
(19) Fibula

(20) Tarsals
(21) Metatarsals
(22) Phalanges

A.

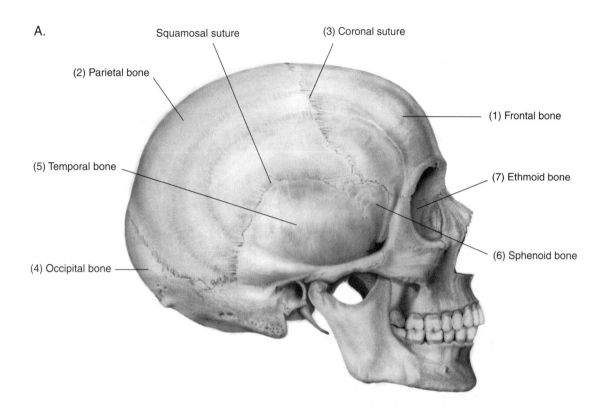

Squamosal suture

(3) Coronal suture

(2) Parietal bone

(1) Frontal bone

(5) Temporal bone

(7) Ethmoid bone

(6) Sphenoid bone

(4) Occipital bone

B.

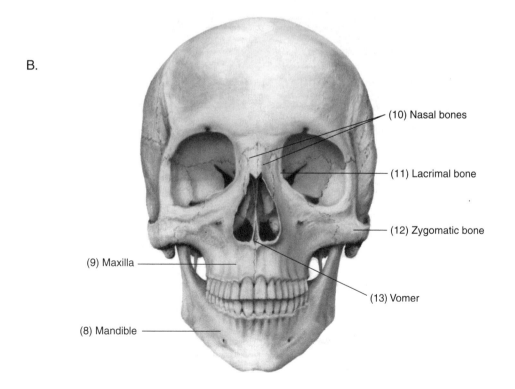

(10) Nasal bones

(11) Lacrimal bone

(12) Zygomatic bone

(9) Maxilla

(13) Vomer

(8) Mandible

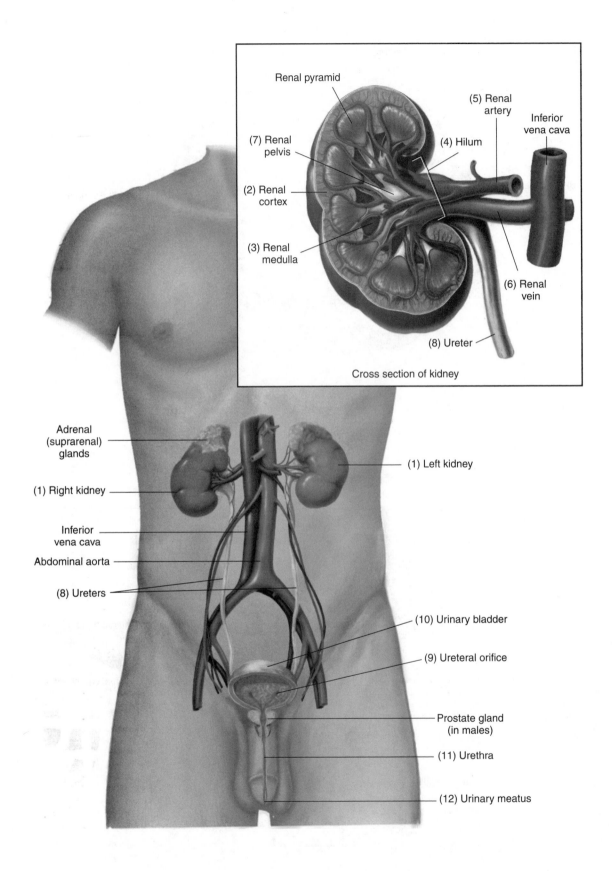

Renal pyramid

(5) Renal artery

Inferior vena cava

(7) Renal pelvis

(4) Hilum

(2) Renal cortex

(3) Renal medulla

(6) Renal vein

(8) Ureter

Cross section of kidney

Adrenal (suprarenal) glands

(1) Left kidney

(1) Right kidney

Inferior vena cava

Abdominal aorta

(8) Ureters

(10) Urinary bladder

(9) Ureteral orifice

Prostate gland (in males)

(11) Urethra

(12) Urinary meatus

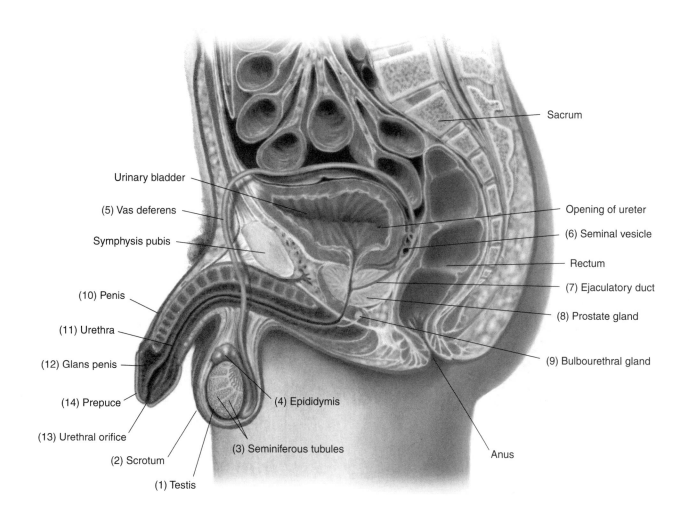

Sacrum

Urinary bladder

(5) Vas deferens

Symphysis pubis

Opening of ureter

(6) Seminal vesicle

Rectum

(7) Ejaculatory duct

(10) Penis

(8) Prostate gland

(11) Urethra

(12) Glans penis

(9) Bulbourethral gland

(14) Prepuce

(13) Urethral orifice

(4) Epididymis

(2) Scrotum

(3) Seminiferous tubules

Anus

(1) Testis

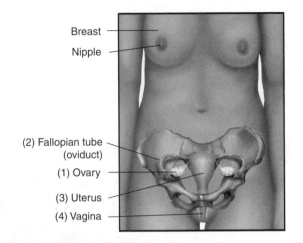

Breast

Nipple

(2) Fallopian tube
(oviduct)

(1) Ovary

(3) Uterus

(4) Vagina

A. Anterior view

Peritoneal
cavity

(1) Ovary

(2) Fallopian tube
(oviduct)

Urinary bladder

Pubis

Urethra

(7) Clitoris

(5) Labia minora

(6) Labia majora

Sacrum

(3) Uterus

Rectum

Cervix

Anus

(4) Vagina

Perineum

(8) Bartholin gland

B. Sagittal section

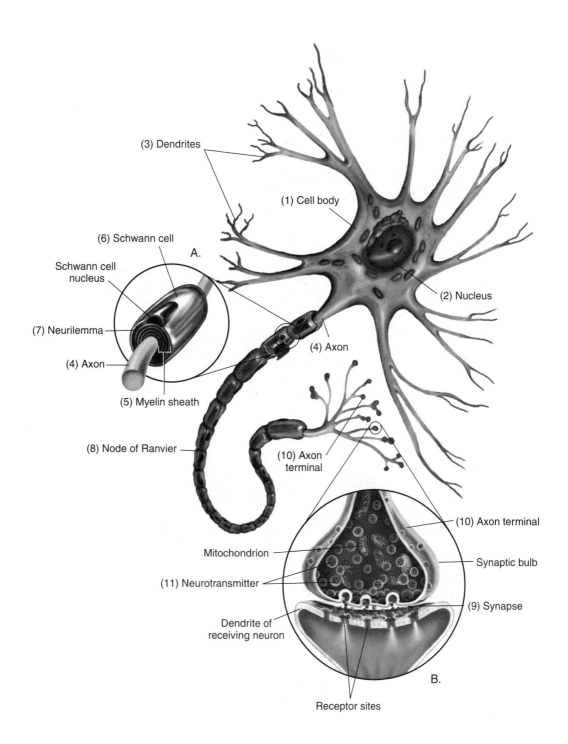

(3) Dendrites

(1) Cell body

(6) Schwann cell

A.

Schwann cell nucleus

(7) Neurilemma

(4) Axon

(5) Myelin sheath

(8) Node of Ranvier

(2) Nucleus

(4) Axon

(10) Axon terminal

(10) Axon terminal

Synaptic bulb

Mitochondrion

(11) Neurotransmitter

(9) Synapse

Dendrite of receiving neuron

B.

Receptor sites

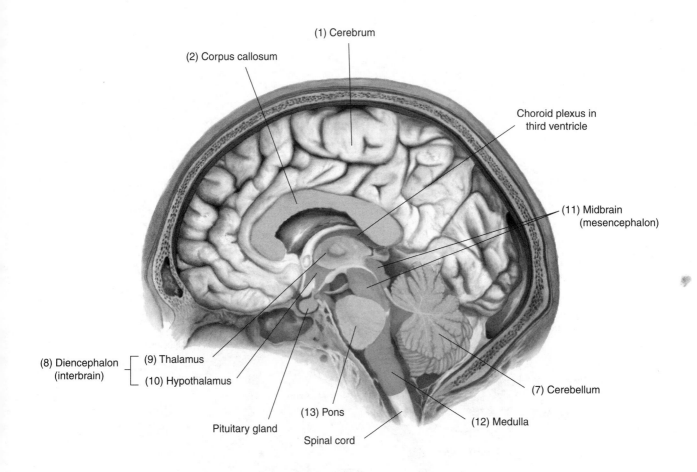

(1) Cerebrum

(2) Corpus callosum

Choroid plexus in
third ventricle

(11) Midbrain
(mesencephalon)

(8) Diencephalon
(interbrain)

(9) Thalamus

(10) Hypothalamus

(7) Cerebellum

Pituitary gland

(13) Pons

(12) Medulla

Spinal cord

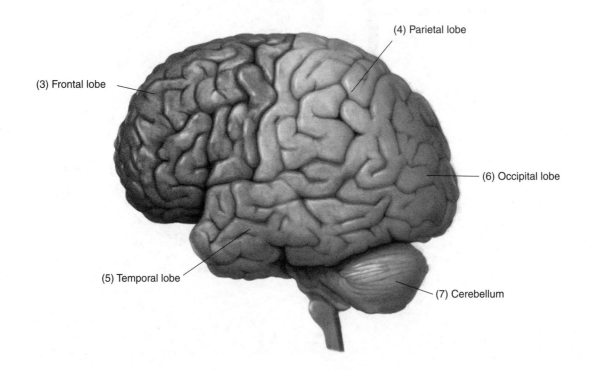

(4) Parietal lobe

(3) Frontal lobe

(6) Occipital lobe

(5) Temporal lobe

(7) Cerebellum

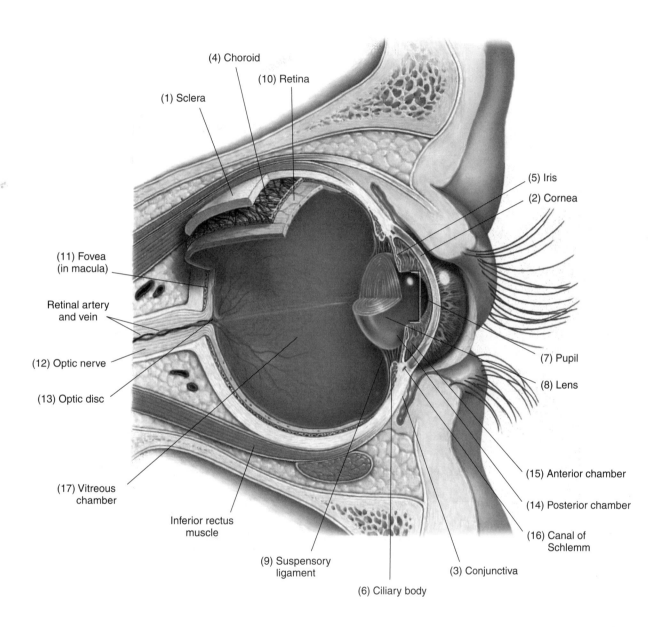

(4) Choroid

(10) Retina

(1) Sclera

(5) Iris

(2) Cornea

(11) Fovea
(in macula)

Retinal artery
and vein

(12) Optic nerve

(7) Pupil

(13) Optic disc

(8) Lens

(15) Anterior chamber

(17) Vitreous
chamber

(14) Posterior chamber

(16) Canal of
Schlemm

Inferior rectus
muscle

(9) Suspensory
ligament

(3) Conjunctiva

(6) Ciliary body

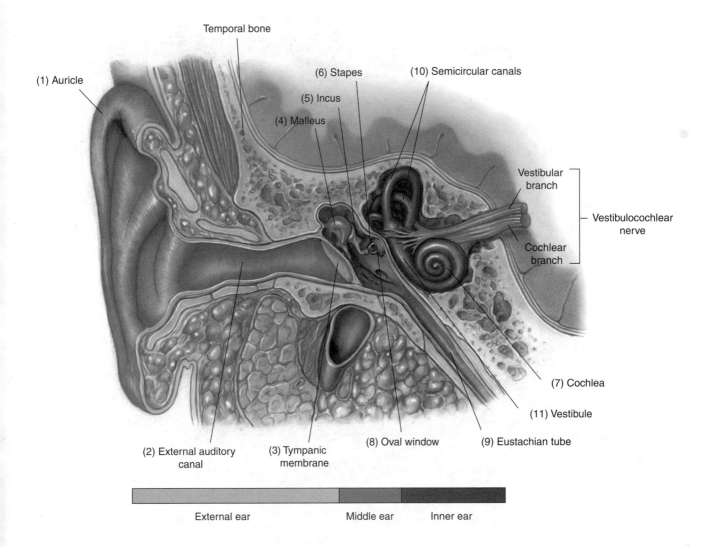

Temporal bone

(1) Auricle

(6) Stapes

(5) Incus

(4) Malleus

(10) Semicircular canals

Vestibular
branch

Vestibulocochlear
nerve

Cochlear
branch

(7) Cochlea

(11) Vestibule

(2) External auditory
canal

(3) Tympanic
membrane

(8) Oval window

(9) Eustachian tube

External ear

Middle ear

Inner ear